TIM STORMS

TOP 50 AT HOME WORKOUTS

TOP 50 EXERCISES YOU CAN DO FROM THE COMFORT OF YOUR HOME

Contents

1

Introduction

I worked out two hours a day when I was in high school. Football and wrestling were a part of every day. Truth be told, the only reason I played sports was because I had five older brothers who played sports. I was more into music myself. Regardless, I wrestled and played football, and wasn't exceptional at either one. I could hold my own, but I had a different calling.

Four days after graduating high school, I moved from Indiana to Oklahoma to join a music group. Actually, with me joining, it became a duo. Nonetheless, we became a group and after much rehearsing we began our first tour that summer in '91. We toured and did shows for a couple months. My workouts came to a screeching halt and I consumed all the fast food over those two months, and I super-sized everything. Maybe it was my 18, almost 19, year old body's metabolism and stress from moving away from home that saved me, but I lost about twenty pounds on that tour. I felt invincible. I felt like I could eat anything without consequence. My brother used to tell me that once I turned thirty, the metabolism goes right out the door. I used to laugh in the face at anything or anyone that would tell me age could play a factor in my body's change over time. Like I said, I felt invincible. So I ate. I ate whatever I wanted, whenever I wanted. So began the trip that got me to where I am now, or where I was five months ago.

Actually, let's backtrack a bit. When I said my workouts came to a screeching halt, they did, but not completely. I would pick up some trips to the gym or the occasional round of push-ups or sit-ups. However, it was certainly not consistent. Rather, it was very sporadic over the years. For some time, after gaining a bit of weight, I was able to take on a couple weeks of push-ups and sit-ups and get right back to my somewhat lean, muscular shape. That was my younger metabolism doing its thing. My brother was right. Once I hit thirty, my metabolism seemed to change, and not for the better. It became increasingly difficult to get into shape as easily as before. Then came forty, then fifty. I went from 172 lbs in high school to 213 lbs at fifty years old. At 5' 10", that's considered overweight. I had a sizable gut on me. By the time I made a decision to get serious about my weight loss, I was 206 lbs. Leading up to fifty years old, I had this recurring thought that I wanted to be ripped at fifty! Actually, for quite some time I haven't been satisfied with how I look. The dad bod creeped up on me and smacked me in the face, and kicked me right in the gut. Clothes I once wore no longer fit. Now that I'm not touring any more, I've been in a regular nine-to-five job wearing dress pants and dress shirts. The waist size gradually got bigger and bigger with seemingly no end in sight. I was extremely uncomfortable in my skin and my clothes, and constantly felt insecure in the way I look. I somehow managed to get down to about 206 lbs. I'm not sure at all how that happened. Maybe it was when I got sick with Covid when that first round hit the world. I did lose some weight that month I was sick. Looking back, I remember not feeling right for quite some time after that. In fact, I remarked several times in the years since then that my body just doesn't feel right.

Who knows what it was, but it all led me to May of 2023. I had had enough of being sick of the way I felt and looked. Lack of energy and stamina were very much a part of my day to day. It was horrible being used to having no energy and no will-power when it came to food intake. Late night snacking was the norm. Who am I kidding?! Late night full-on meals, then snacking and/or dessert were the norm. I had had enough. Hello breaking point. Being ripped at fifty was still on my mind, but getting healthy was at the forefront. In my endless scrolling on social media (yes it's a pandemic of epic proportions that has taken over the world) I came across an app which shall remain nameless. This particular app opened my eyes to my relationship with food. Thus began my journey of eating what I need and with purpose, and exercising. When I started on May 20th of this year (my 28 year wedding anniversary, by the way) I was right about 206 lbs. Now I am down to 176.2 lbs as I write this. It's been a combination of a new relationship with food and exercise that has gotten me to where I am now. I'm not finished yet. I may be 51, but my "ripped at 50" has become ripped in my 50's. Actually, I'm gunning for 51. Which leads me to what's to come in this book. I'd like to lay out the top 50 at home exercises or workouts to help you kickstart your own journey of health and being comfortable in your skin and the way you look and feel. Let's get started.

2

Chapter 1

WHY AT HOME WORKOUTS?

If your story is similar to mine, you have reached your breaking point. That point where you say, enough is enough. I have to do something about the way I look and feel. Which has led you to your inspiration to change. The inspiration will be different on a personal level for everyone, but listen to that inspiration. Your inspiration will lead you to a decision to change. That decision to change should lead you to a plan of action. Lay out your goals. What do you want to accomplish? How do you want to get there? Once you have a plan, COMMIT to your plan. Stick to the process. If you can make a commitment to your plan of change, you can succeed at this.

And whatever you do, do not make this part of your New Year's resolution. Most New Year's resolutions end in failure. Why? Because most people think about their resolutions before the end of the year and say, for my New Year's resolution, I'm going to do this or that. So they have from December whatever the date is to the end of the year to keep up with their bad habit, whatever that may be. They keep feeding the bad habit with every intention to stop cold turkey at the beginning of the year. This is not a productive way to stop a bad habit and change. If you want to change, it starts now. If you want to change, don't tell everyone you plan to do it on such and such day. Just quietly begin now. People will see the change. People will be inspired by the change and growth. Someone very close to me was inspired on some level to make a change after seeing changes begin in me.

If you are like me, working out at the gym is not really your cup of tea. I prefer to work out in the comfort of my own home without needless distractions and the smells of countless others working out. At home workouts offer you the opportunity to do it at your own pace without someone else staring you down until you give up the bench press or leg curl machine. That's another thing. Working out at home affords you the opportunity to be creative in how you accomplish your goals, without having to use all the gym equipment. The only thing I use besides my own body weight is workout tubes with handles.

A great advantage to working out at home instead of the gym is cost, or lack thereof. Unless you decide to purchase your own workout equipment, which can cost anywhere from under a hundred bucks to several thousand dollars depending on what you invest in, working out at home can be absolutely free. No having to sell a kidney to afford a gym membership. It's free! Also, your time is your own. Work out whenever you want. No commute times back and forth to the gym. That alone can take a huge chunk out of your day. Another advantage of working out at home instead of the gym is the only person you are comparing yourself to at home is you. When you're at the gym, it can be easy to compare yourself to others, even on a subliminal level. At home, you compare yourself to yourself. That's it. Unless of course you're flipping through muscle or fitness magazines. How many of us have compared ourselves to famous celebrities who are completely ripped with zero body fat? I think we all have done this on some level. Or at least noticed the celebrity physique and thought how cool it would be to be that ripped. I say all that to say, it can be intimidating being at the gym and seeing people who are much further along in their journey than you are in yours. Everyone is on a different journey. Some further along than others. That's okay. We all started at different times, so extending grace where appropriate is a must. Some people will be further along in their journey than you are in yours, and some will not yet have started their journey to a better self. Extend grace. Be someone's inspiration. That said, working out at home is certainly less intimidating than working out at the gym.

3

Chapter 2

EATING HAS CONSEQUENCES

Everything you do has consequences. It's amazing how the dad bod creeps up on you. It doesn't happen by accident. It's a calculated effort, whether you realize it or not. Every last bit of food you ingest will either have a positive or negative consequence. Unless you throw pickles in there. Completely free of calories. But since we can't live on pickles, yes, everything you eat will have some sort of consequence, even if it's not readily visible. Think of how long it takes for all those pounds to accumulate. For some, it can take years. For others, maybe it only took you a year or less to gain fifty pounds. Stress, overeating, or even health conditions can lead to excessive weight gain. If you are one who suffers from certain health conditions that make it difficult to lose weight, I am not a health professional and have no certifications that empower me to be able to advise you on the correct path to take. Please seek the help of a medical professional. For all others, I am speaking from personal experience and hope to impart to you some words of wisdom and most of all, encouragement and specific exercises that will help you on your own journey to reach your ultimate goals.

But before we get to those specific workouts, have you heard the term you are what you eat? It's true. Everything you ingest will manifest itself in your body as what it is. If you ingest nothing but fatty foods with tons of processed sugar, guess what, it will manifest itself as fat in your body. Pounds upon pounds will develop and grow over the weeks, months, and years until you see a picture of you that someone took and you realize you're the one with the big gut in the picture. Really?! Is this how everyone sees me? If you regularly eat more than a serving at a time, the pounds will pile on. Most restaurants serve meals that are far greater than a serving size, in terms of daily recommended calorie intake. Some are two to three times a serving size! Which brings me to my next point.

Aside from sticking to eating just the recommended serving size of whatever food I happen to be eating at the time, which is one of the most important things that has helped me lose close to thirty pounds in the last five months, is paying attention to caloric density. Eating foods with a focus on caloric density, or lack thereof, is key to maintaining or even losing weight. Caloric density has to do with how many calories a food has in direct proportion to how much it weighs. Choosing foods like vegetables, fish, lean meats, egg whites, and whole grain breads, etc, that have a low caloric density will make you feel more full or satiated without making you feel bloated and adding on the pounds. Foods with high caloric density, such as anything with processed sugar, desserts like cake or donuts, greasy foods with oils, chips, cheeseburger and fries, etc, will most certainly have you on a path to putting on the pounds and attaining the dad bod you always wanted.

Timing your meals is very important as well. I'm not saying you have to eat every meal at certain times. Listen to your body. Your body will tell you when you are hungry. Now, there's a difference between your stomach telling you you're hungry and your brain telling you you're hungry. I would suggest you read up on the psychology of eating to attain a deeper understanding of how our brains work when it comes to feeding our faces and bellies. Again, listen to your body. Your body will tell you when it's time to eat. The difficulty can come when determining when it's time to stop eating. If you want to lose the pounds, I would suggest setting a time each evening, preferably at least two to three hours before bedtime, to stop eating. If you eat a meal right before you go to bed, your body is less likely to respond in a positive way. This can make it more difficult for your body to digest the food you eat. Also, eating right before bedtime can often cause acid reflux, which can lead to a difficult night's sleep. Lack of rest can cause lack of energy. Lack of energy can cause... and so on and so on. It's a snowball effect.

It is entirely possible to lose weight and maintain that weight loss on a sustainable level by paying attention to eating foods with a focus on caloric density. However, for those that desire a more fit or lean appearance, I would suggest adding exercise or working out to your daily routine. In the next chapter, I'll outline my top fifty at home workouts/exercises that will, when used properly, get you on the road to a fit physique. Combining exercise with a sensible eating routine for your age, height, weight, etc. will be the most sustainable way to get the pounds off and keep them off. Please consult a doctor or nutritionist for guidance on your specific dietary needs and what exercises would be safe for you.

4

Chapter 3

HOME WORKOUTS

Keep in mind, these exercises are not listed in any particular order in terms of favorite to least favorite, or most effective to least effective. I will group them according to type of exercise and what areas they target the most. The first grouping will be exercises that are geared toward using your own body weight as the resistance. The second grouping will be for those who have resistance bands or resistance tubes with handles. All the exercises listed will be exercises you can do from the comfort of your home. Again, please consult a doctor to determine if any of the following exercises are safe for you. I am not a licensed trainer and speak only from personal experience with exercise and working out, so take what I say and consult a professional to avoid injury. And we begin.

Number 1. Wide Arm Push Ups

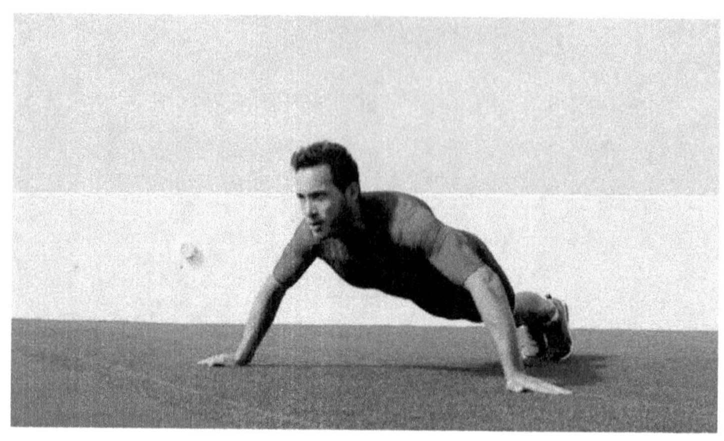

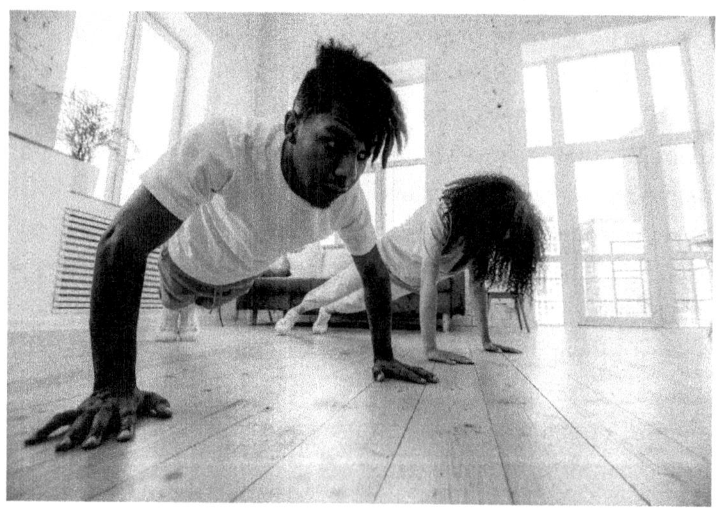

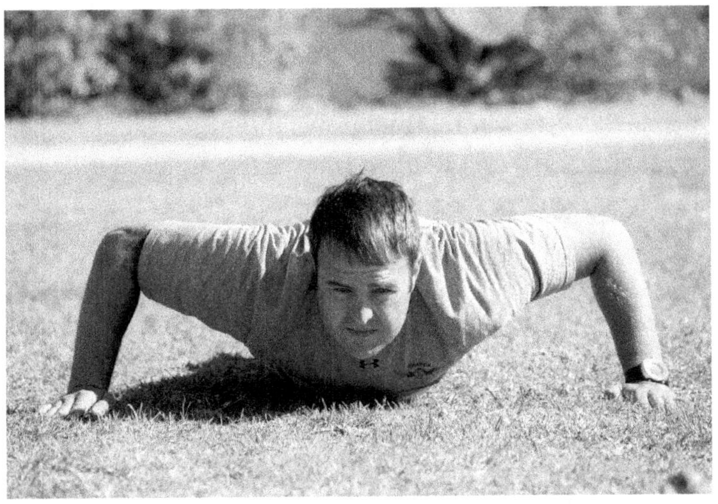

When doing these wide arm pushups, you want to be careful not to strain your shoulders.You can experiment with placement when doing these and other forms of push ups. By placement I mean where your hands are in relation to where your head and shoulders are. If you shift your head/body forward or back (closer to being in line with your hands vs positioning your head out in front of where your hands align), depending on what is more comfortable, you will target certain muscles with a bit more precision. Like I said, just experiment with it. The key to successful exercise, outside of a balanced diet, is consistency. Working out one day a week is certainly better than nothing at all, however, working out at least three or four days a week will offer you the opportunity to see more measurable results!

If you are a beginner to exercise, just do as many of these as is comfortable, even if it's not a whole pushup. You've got to start somewhere. The point is, you are starting. Just keep going. Do one today, maybe two tomorrow, three the next day. Build your way up to where you can do reps of five or ten. Maybe even fifteen or twenty or more.

If you are not a stranger to exercise and can do reps of ten or twenty at a time, it's good to alternate types of pushups between ab exercises. I like to start with Wide Arm Push Ups, move to crunches, then on to standard Shoulder Width Push Ups, crunches again, Tricep Push Ups, and one more round of crunches. This gives my arms a bit of a rest between sets.

Technique is very important, and more important than speed, if you want to achieve optimum results. Be sure to keep your back as straight as you can and head looking forward. Dropping down with each push up should result in your chest touching the floor. For some of us, the first thing to hit the floor will be your stomach. That's okay. Just go down as far as you can so your arms get the proper cycle of release and extension.

Number 2. Shoulder Width Push Ups

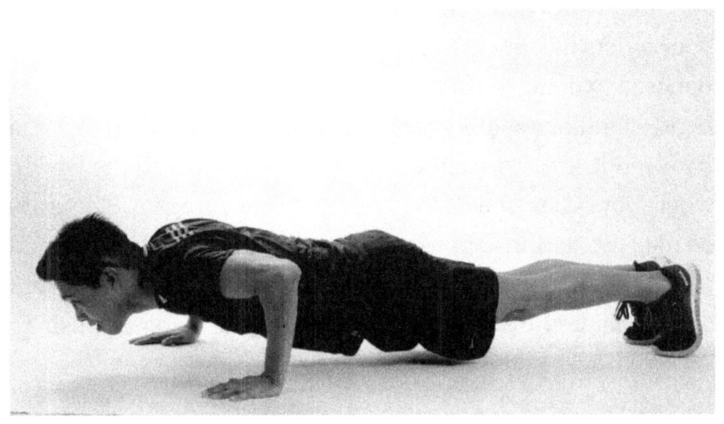

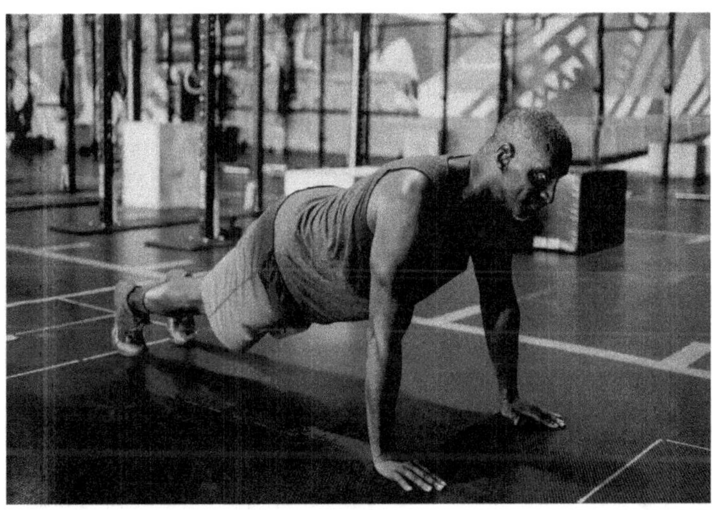

These are your standard push ups. Make sure your hands are

shoulder width apart. If you have carpal tunnel or issues with your wrists like me, it helps to do push ups with your fists, as opposed to doing them with hands flat on the floor. Keep your hands shoulder width apart and perpendicular to the floor as shown in the picture above. Again, come down all the way to where your chest meets the floor and back up again. There are so many variations of push ups. To spice it up a bit, you could elevate your feet on a chair or exercise step. This would work your shoulders and pecs a bit more than your standard push up.

Number 3. Tricep Push Up

17

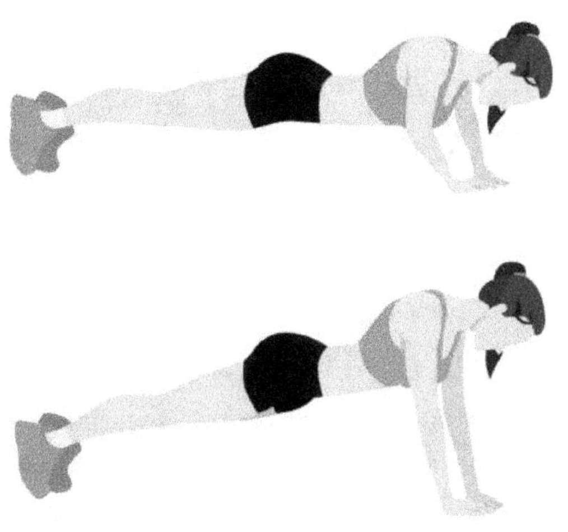

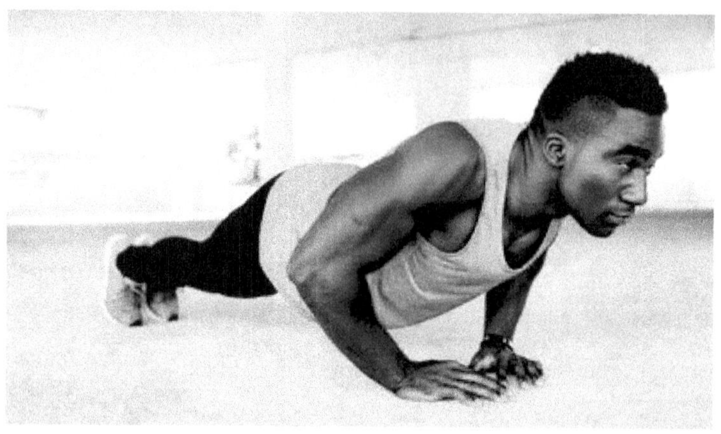

The tricep push up is very effective at working your tricep muscles. You need to make sure your positioning is correct so as not to cause injury. If you have shoulder issues, approach this exercise with caution. As with all exercise, it's a good idea to stretch prior to any exercise. Proper placement for optimum results for the tricep push up, also known as the triangle or diamond push up, is found by placing your hands in such a way as to make a triangle or diamond shape. Keeping this shape, begin your push ups with your chest meeting the tops of your hands, and back up again. Similar to the wide arm push ups, you can experiment with placement of your head/body in relation to where your hands are.

Number 4. Negative Push Ups

This will work with all forms of push ups and numerous other exercises as well. When doing a negative push up, you must concentrate on proper form for optimum results. Push up, then when dropping back down, go down slowly to a count to five to eight seconds with each rep.

Number 5. Ankle Touch Crunches

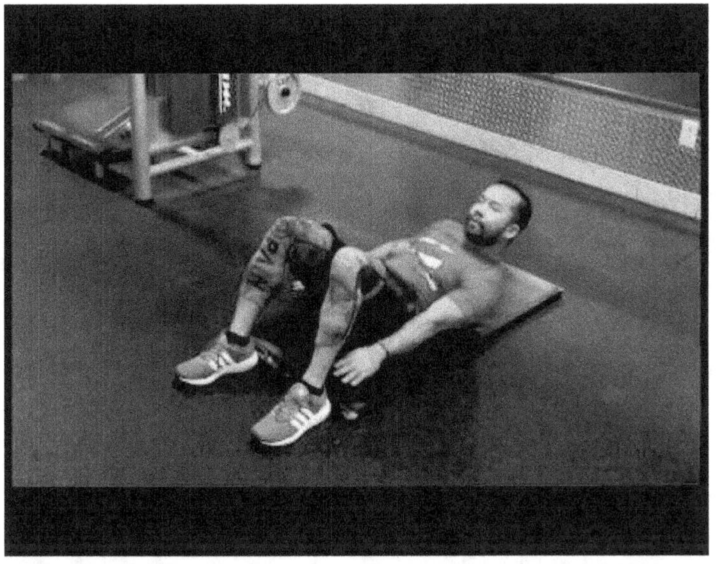

Where crunches alone do not get rid of a spare tire or beer belly, they are an effective way to build tone and definition in your abs. All the crunches in the world won't do you a bit of good if your diet is out of control, so mind your diet along with exercise to obtain optimum results.

Laying with your back on the floor and your knees up, alternate touches to each ankle or heel while keeping your head and shoulders off the floor. There is a noticeable difference when reaching for the ankle as opposed to the heel. You can actually reach beyond your ankle or heel to a point in space just beyond your shin. If you want to put this into a workout, you could do sets of each where with one set you reach to your heel, another you reach to your ankle, and lastly, you reach just beyond your shin. You could even combine all of these into each set; heel/heel, ankle/ankle, shin/shin, past your leg/past your leg and start over again.

Number 6. Cross Arm Crunches

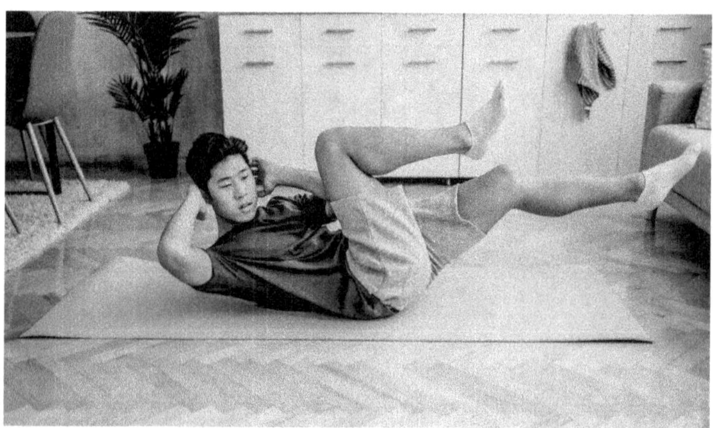

Rather than your typical up-down, up-down of the traditional crunch, this crunch variation employs a twist. As seen in the picture, in tandem with your crunch motion, you bring your knees, one at a time toward your chest. From there, it's left elbow to right knee alternating from right elbow to left knee. It's like a bike pedaling motion with a twist of the upper torso. Now, it would be easy to speed through this exercise for maximum reps, but that may be counter productive. For optimum results with the Cross Arm Crunches, go at a slow to moderate pace focusing on, and engaging the muscles you feel this exercise affecting. It also works to employ this exercise in between push up sets.

Number 7. Cross Crunches

Cross Crunches are similar to Cross Arm Crunches, with two marked differences. Number one, you will keep your knees up with feet on the floor. Number two, you will move elbows to opposite legs, but you will extend your arm to touch the outside of your knee, leg or calf. You can actually use all three positions; right hand to outside of left knee, left hand to outside of right knee, then right hand to outside of left thigh, left hand to outside of right thigh, then right hand to outside of left calf, left hand to outside of right calf. Be sure to keep your shoulders off the floor as much as possible with this exercise for the best results.

Number 8. Reverse Crunches

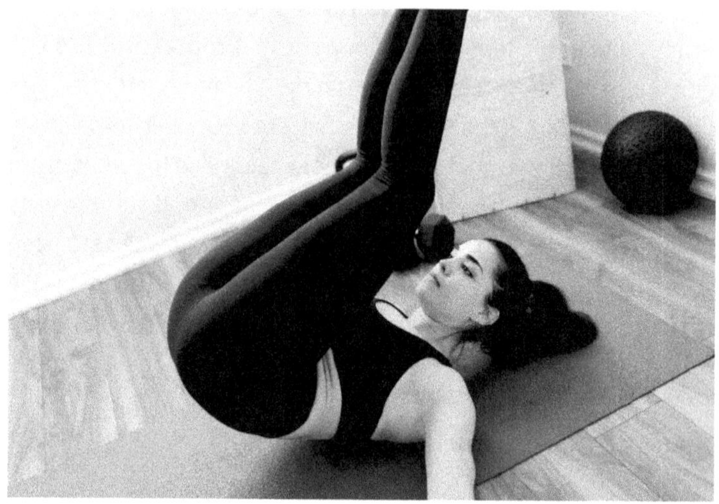

 If you happen to have back issues, or a medical condition that may impede your workout or may be exacerbated by this or any of the exercises in this book, please consult a physician before proceeding. As someone with back issues, this particular exercise is one with which I have to be cautious.

Laying flat on the floor with arms spread wide for stability and control, lift your legs up until they are ninety degrees to your torso. With your legs in the air, lift your butt off the floor, engaging your core muscles. You can then bring your legs either back down to where they are flat on the floor, or just to the ninety degree mark. Try both ways and notice the difference in the muscles at work. From there you can decide which way works better for you.

Number 9. Side Planks (with hip raise and leg to chest)

23

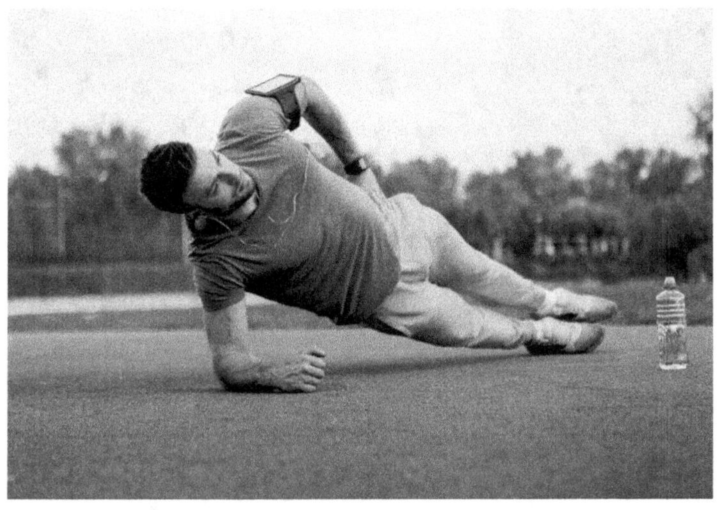

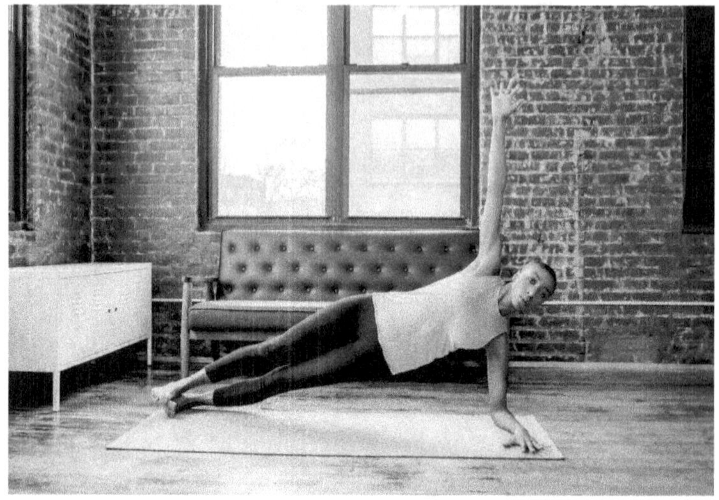

 The pictures show a basic side plank. It's self explanatory in terms of what the exercise is. You put yourself in the position as seen in the pictures, and sit there. Lay there? Whatever it is, I have added a couple things to this particular plank. First position is the basic plank. Second position is bringing your free (top) arm down in a body-twisting motion toward your elbow that is on the floor and back to first position. Third position is raising your hip to the ceiling and back down to the first position. Fourth position is bringing your top leg to your chest in order to engage your core muscles, and back to first position, then repeat all positions. I do about five of these, then switch to the other side. Alternating these between sets of push ups is very effective in terms of giving yourself a rest from that particular exercise while you're doing another exercise.

Number 10. Leg Raise into Reverse Lunge

25

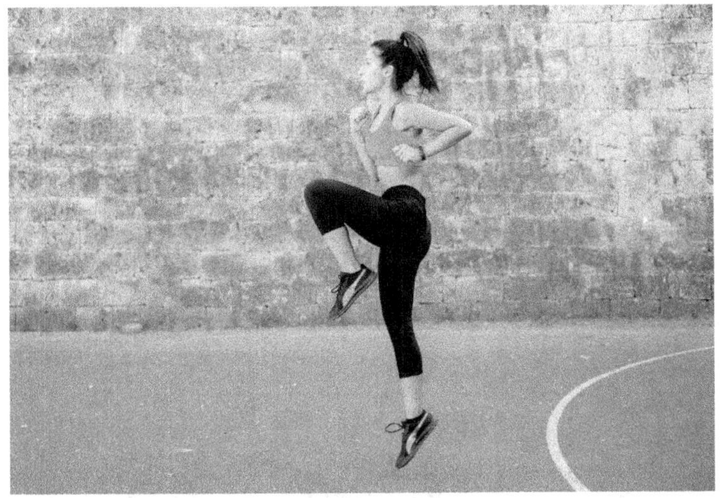

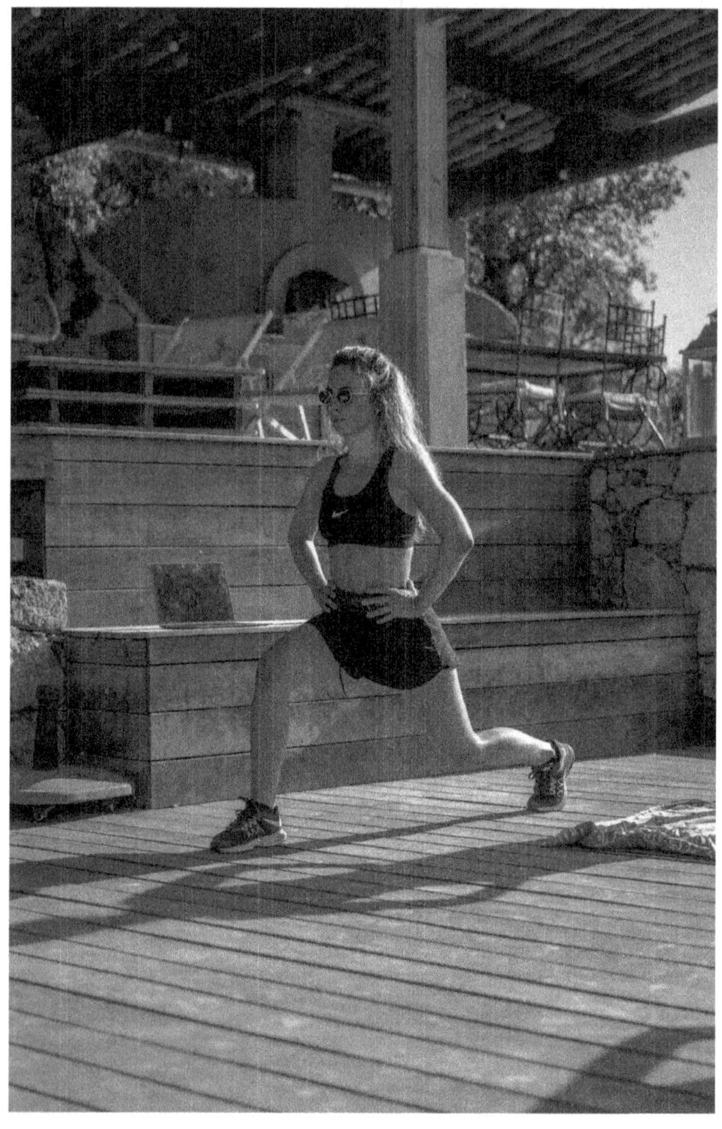

This exercise takes a bit of getting used to in terms of keeping your balance. It will engage your core, as well as work your quads and hamstrings. You begin in a standing position. Kick one leg up toward your chest while keeping your other leg on the ground/floor. While doing this, engage your abs. The picture shows the model jumping up. This is something you can do, if you choose, but I find I am more able to engage my ab muscles by keeping my foot planted. After kicking up, bring your leg back down without planting your foot. Keep your leg in motion and let it swing through and behind you to the point of a reverse lunge, as seen in the picture. After a set on one side, switch to the other and begin the process again.

Number 11. Wall Sit

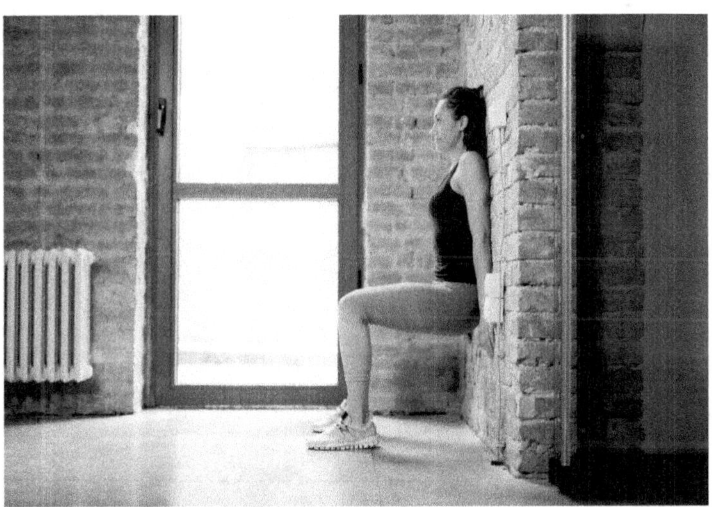

Wall sitting brings back torturous memories of wrestling practice in the 8th grade. As part of our workout, we would do wall sits, but our coach was really serious about wall sitting. That's putting it lightly. One practice, we did wall sits for thirty minutes. Pure torture. My legs were burning so bad by the end of the session, I could hardly walk. The entire process of wall sitting is exactly what you see in the picture. "Sitting" on the wall with no chair or anything to support you, except your back up against the wall. When you do this exercise, start in small timed increments and work your way up. You may even have to start with ten or fifteen seconds and work your way up from there. Try to improve your time to where you are able to sit there for minutes at a time. Talk about a burn!

Number 12. Squats

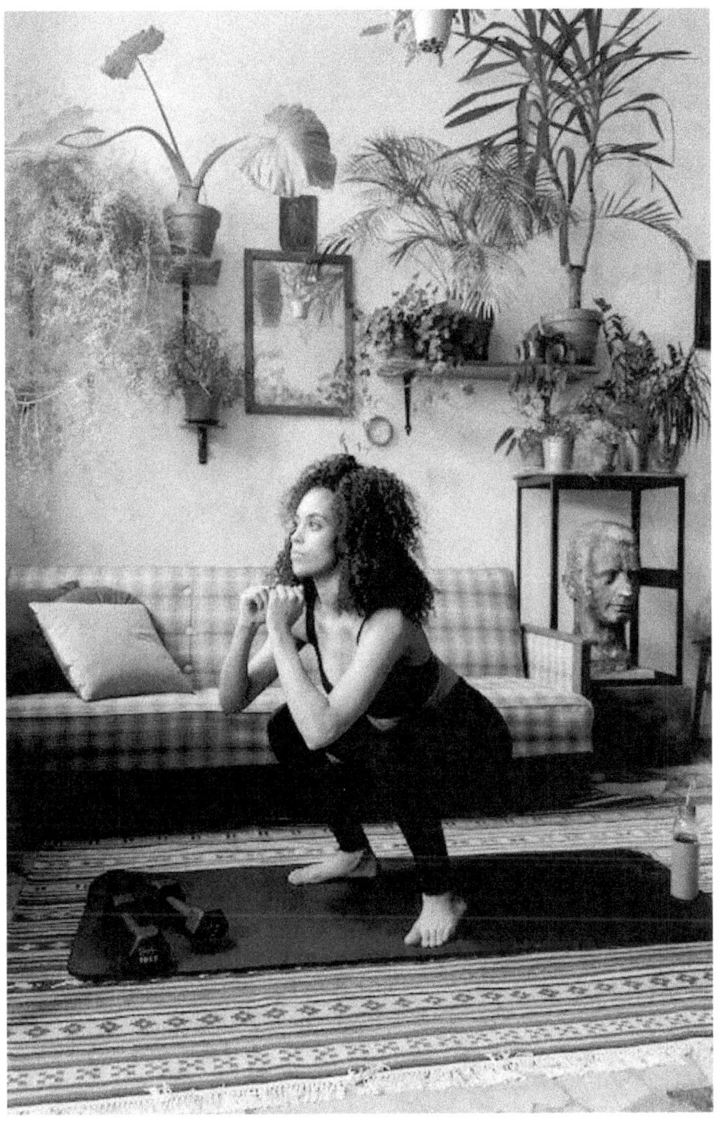

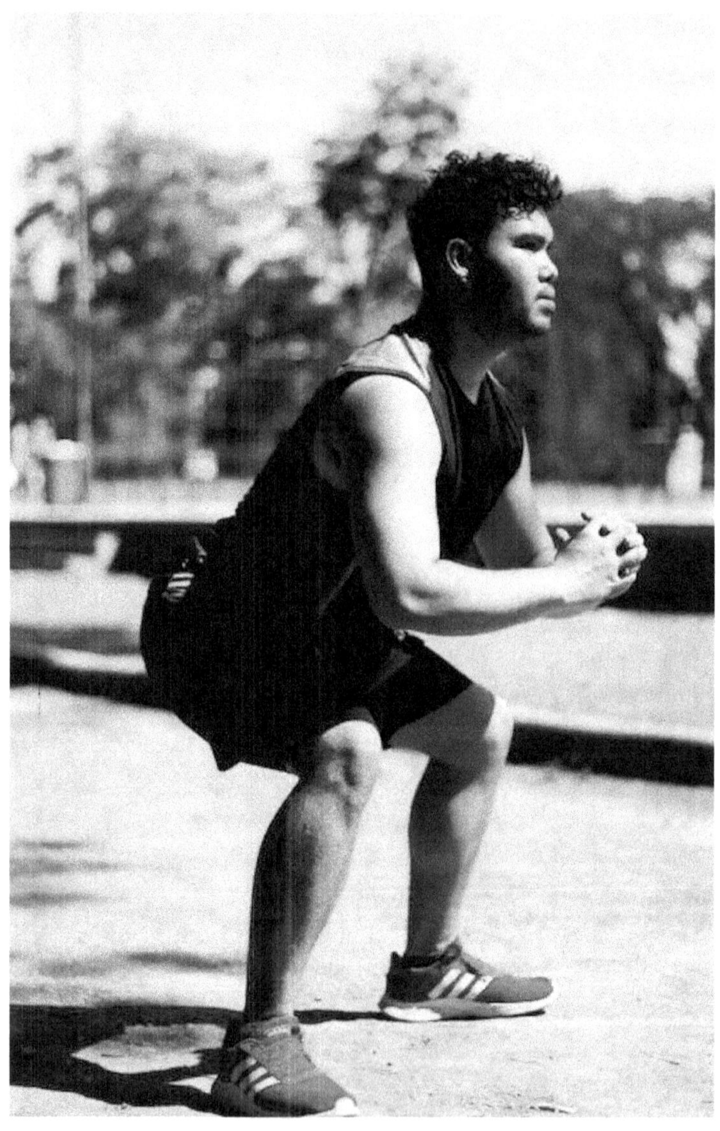

I always hated leg day. But here we are. Another exercise that works your legs. Yay. If you want to have a strong upper body, it makes zero sense to not have a strong base. You need a strong core and strong legs to support whatever you have going on up top. A good, solid foundation is key. That goes for just about anything in life.

A regular squat routine can certainly help you lay that firm foundation you need for the ripped upper body you hope to attain. Technique is key here. It's not just simply squatting down and back up again. You want to keep your back straight and looking forward. It helps to bring your hands together in front of you with arms bent, like in the pictures. From a standing position with legs about shoulder width apart, squat into a seated position, then back up again. Squats should not be rushed. You want to feel and engage the muscles you are working.

Number 13. Plank Leg Lifts

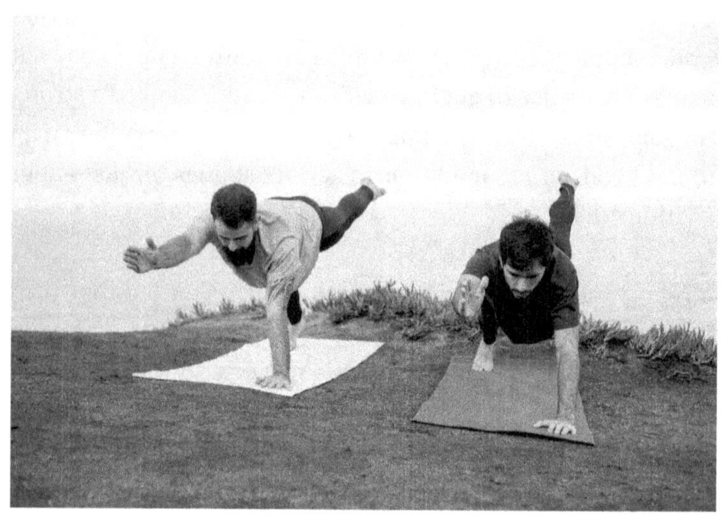

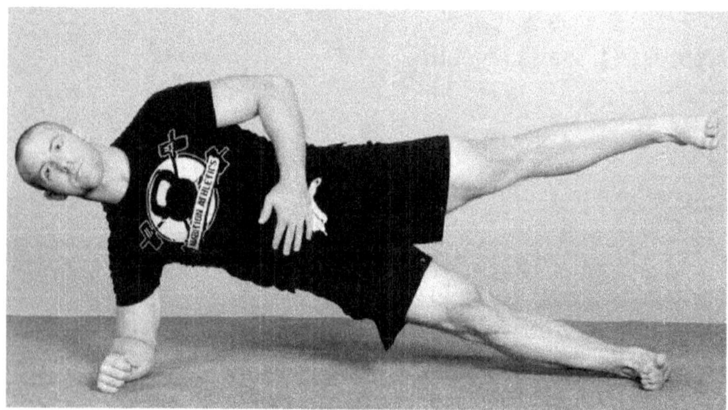

We previously covered side planks with a couple additions to the exercise. These particular planks, be it the traditional plank or side plank, just add a simple leg lift to the exercise. The side plank with leg lift is the simpler of the two. From your side plank position, simply raise your free leg and back down again. Do several reps and switch to the other side.

The plank in the first picture is a bit more involved, at least in terms of balance. In the up position of a push up, lift the left leg and the right arm at the same time and hold this position. After you feel like you're about to collapse (just kidding - don't do that) switch to the other side and repeat.

Number 14. Bicycle Crunch

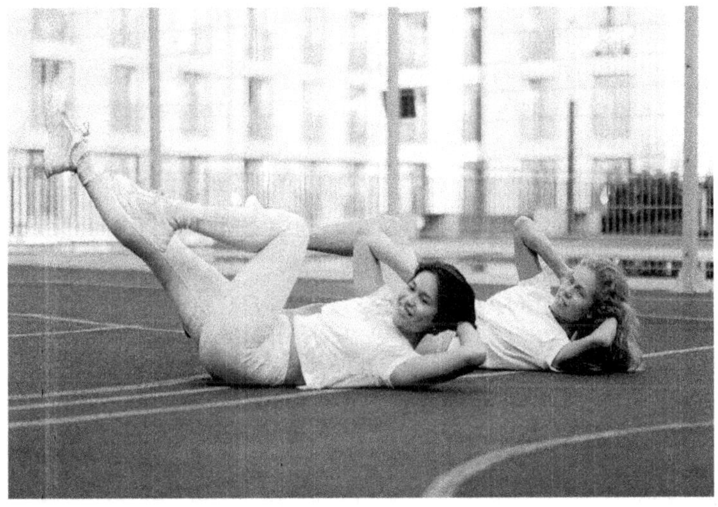

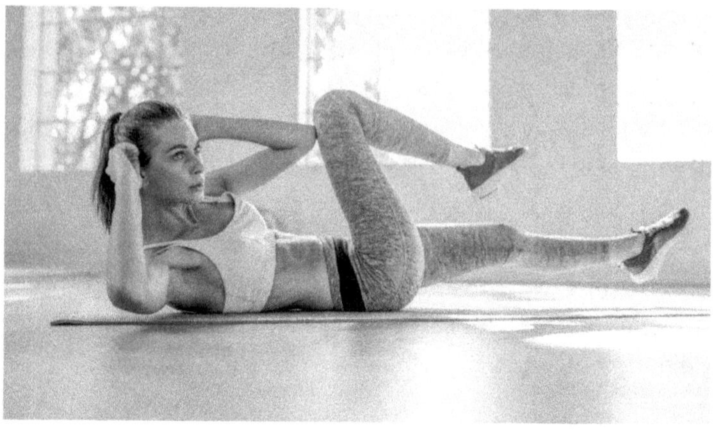

Bicycle Crunches are similar to the crunches previously mentioned, but without any variation to the exercise. Keeping your head and shoulders off the floor, kick legs up one at a time while touching the opposite elbow to your knee. Left elbow to right knee, and right elbow to left knee, back and forth. Feel the core muscles being activated and concentrate on those. Keep them engaged throughout the exercise.

Number 15. Reverse Bicycle

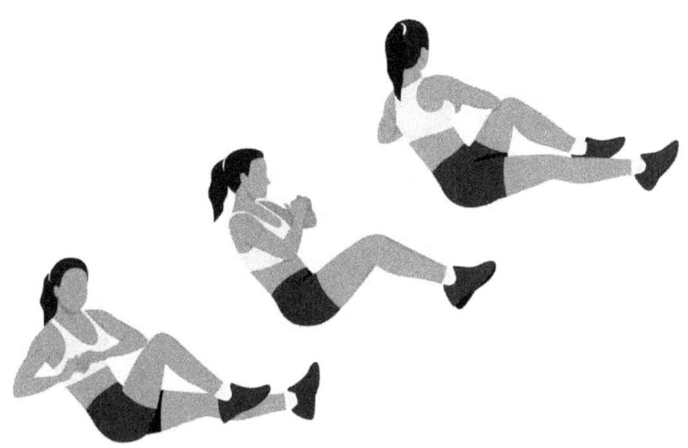

For the Reverse Bicycle, you start with a v sit position, then with a motion as if you are pedaling a bicycle backwards, move your legs back and forth in that manner. The picture shows a torso twist being done, but that is a level of difficulty you can opt for at your discretion.

Number 16. Diver's Push Ups

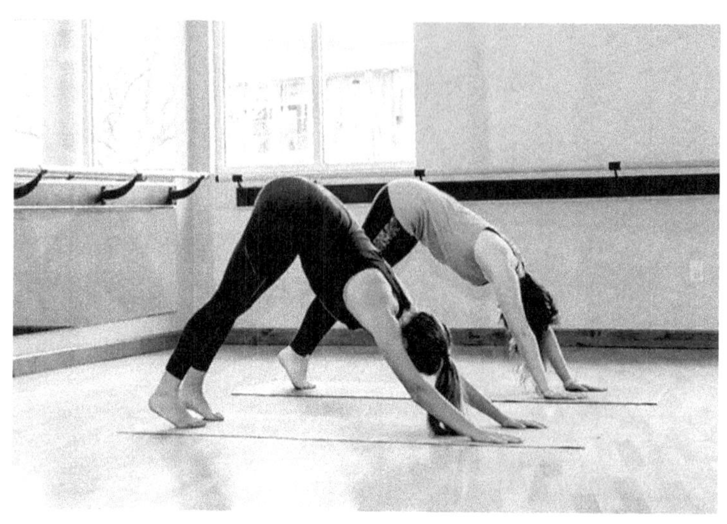

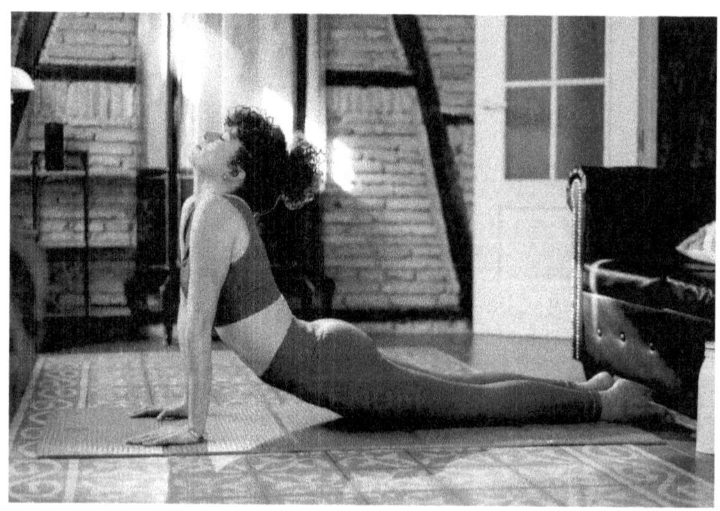

Begin the Diver's Push Ups with only feet and hands on the floor, with butt up in the air making a triangle with the floor. Slowly with your head, dip your head down to the floor as if to draw a J shape with your head, ending with legs on the floor, pushing your upper body upward and extending your arms fully and firmly planted on the floor with your head reaching for the ceiling.

Number 17. Burpees

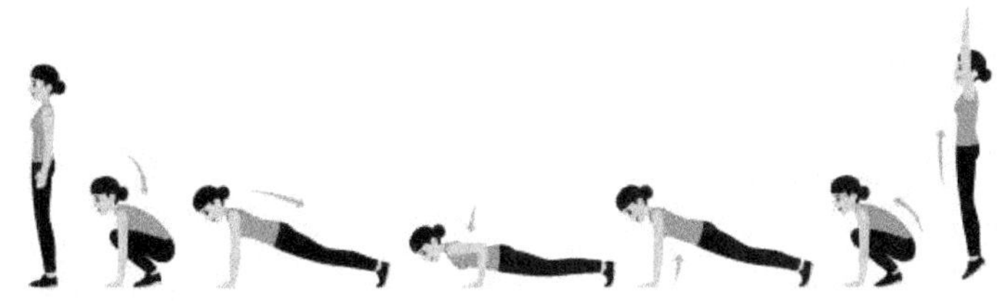

 The picture above speaks for itself. These really get your heart pumping. Again, consult your physician before attempting strenuous exercises such as this.

Number 18. Mountain Climbers

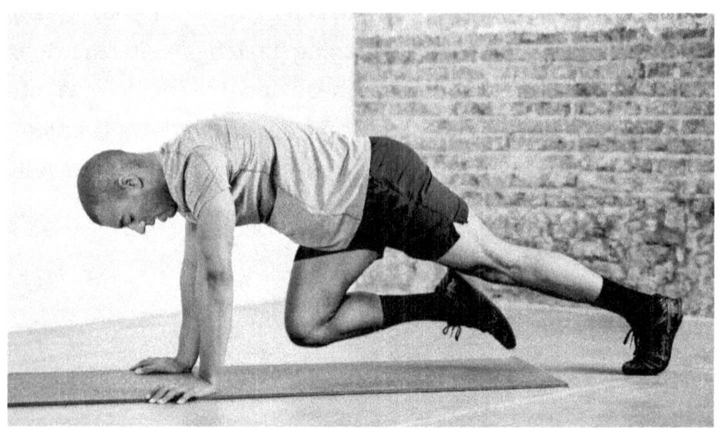

In a push up position, alternate your legs back and forth as if you are climbing a mountain.

Number 19. Hip Raises

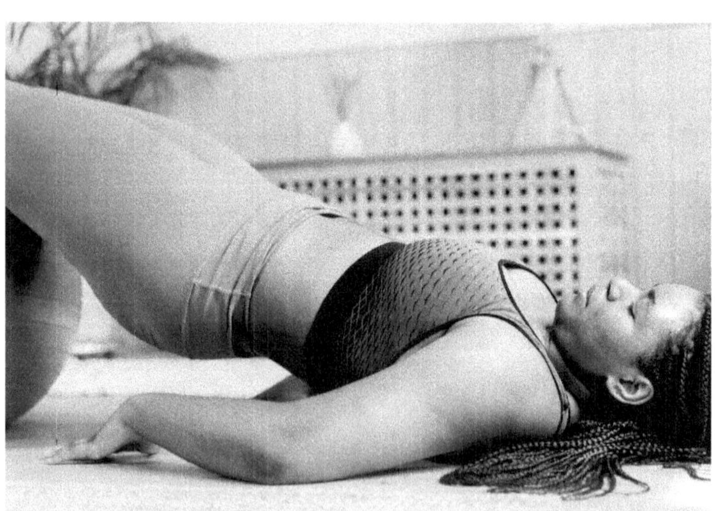

The picture shows this exercise being done with an exercise ball. You can also do this using a chair or from the edge of a couch, as well as using just your bent leg to be able to raise your hips. The idea is to elevate your legs, then raise your hips from the floor upward.

Number 20. Single Leg Hip Raises

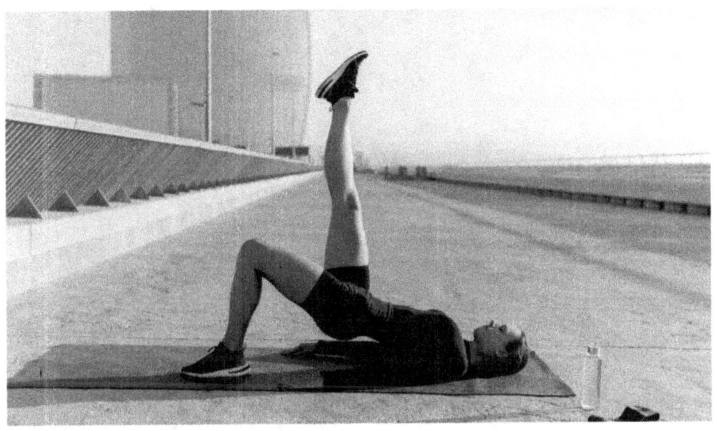

This employs the same principles as the traditional hip raises. The difference is you point one leg upward, or at least as upward as you can get, while raising your hips.

Number 21. Side Plank Leg Lifts

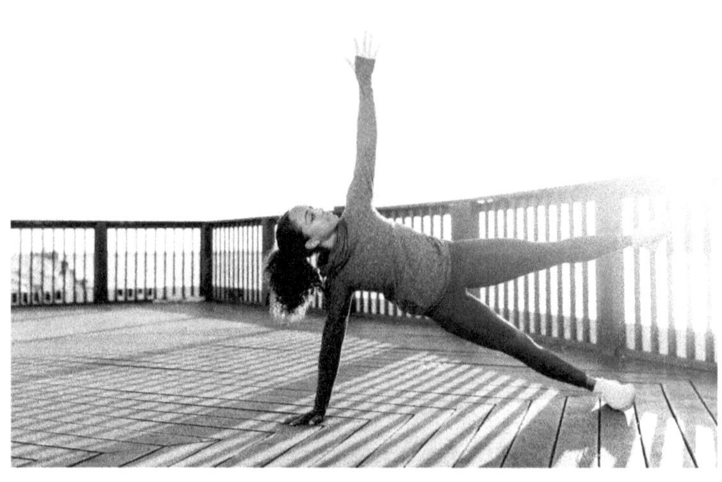

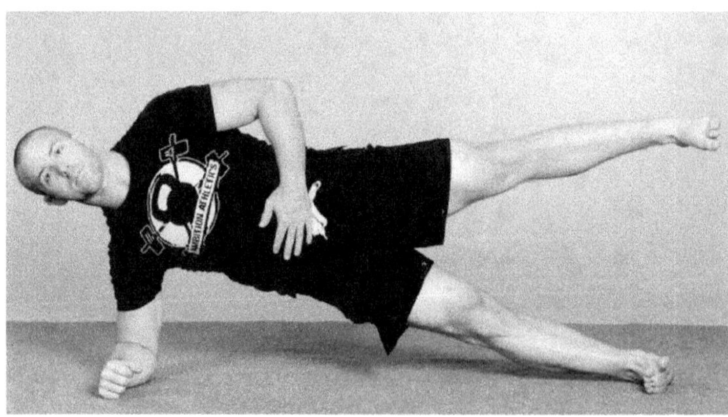

This is a simple side plank with the added leg lift. Do however many reps work for you and switch to the other side and do the same.

Number 22. Tricep Dips (with steps or chair)

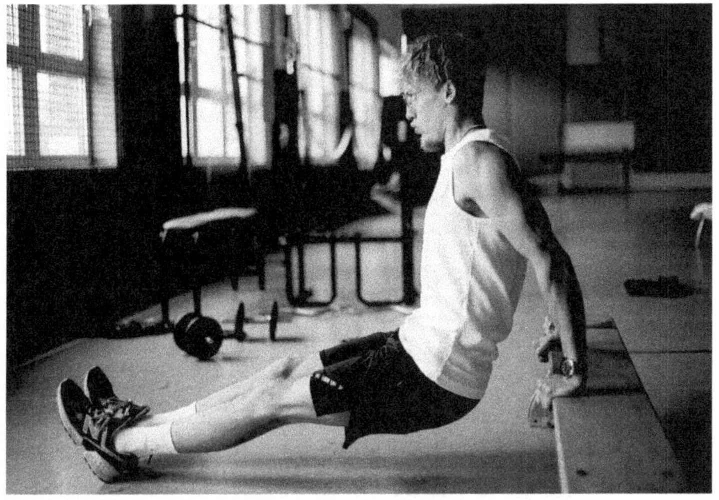

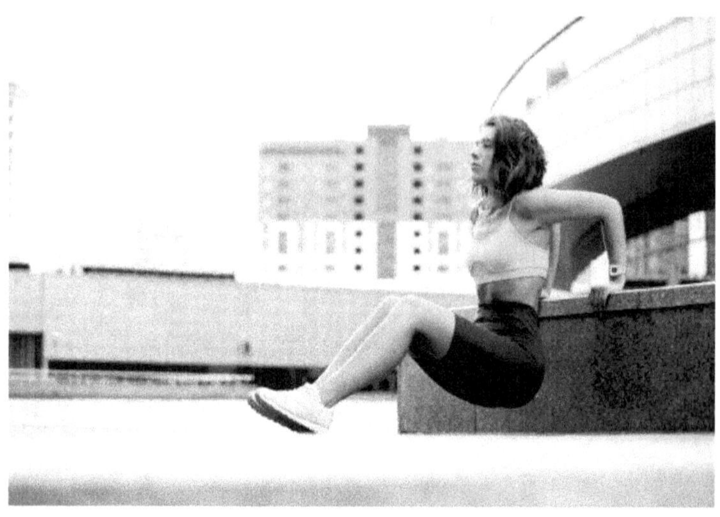

 If you have shoulders that are not in the best shape, be careful with this exercise. It can definitely strain your shoulders. This is meant to work your triceps. It can be done with a retaining wall, chair, or exercise steps. Start in an upward position and lower your body enough that your arm creates a ninety degree angle, upper arm to forearm, and repeat.

Number 23. Tricep Dips on floor

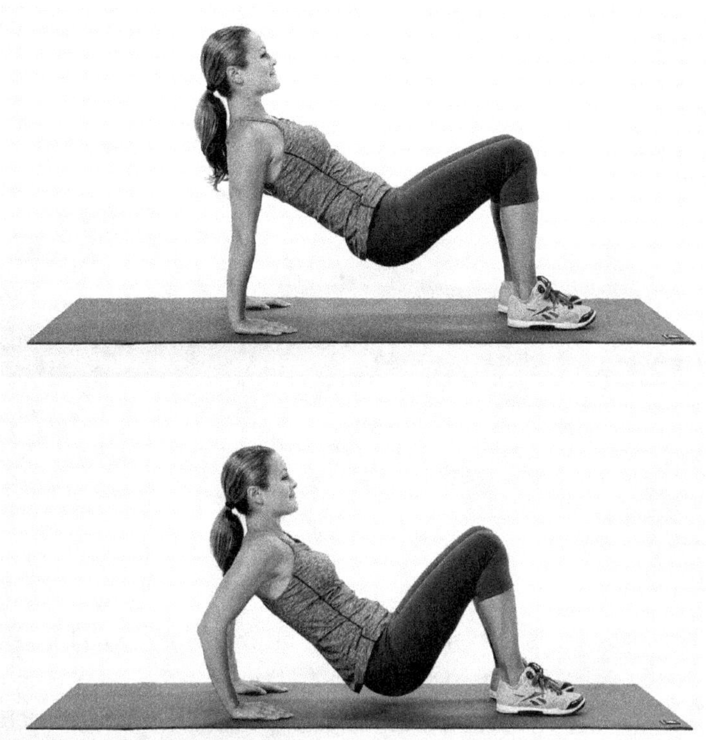

This is the same method as the tricep dips with a chair or wall, but obviously without the chair or wall. You can try each and see which one is more effective for you.

Number 24. Twisted Mountain Climber

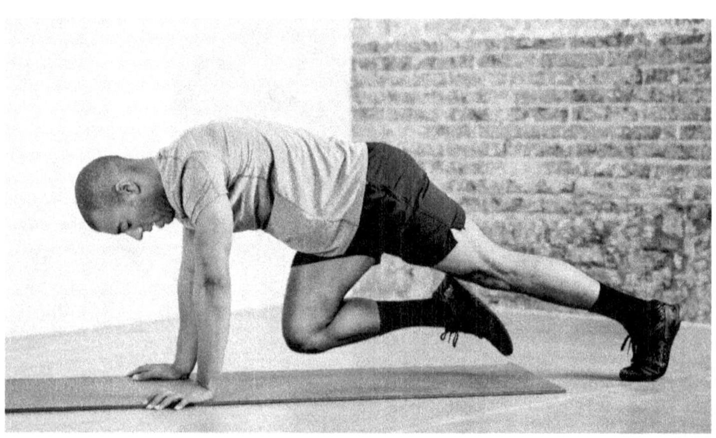

This exercise is the same as the traditional mountain climber, except you will cross your knees to the opposite side of your body. Aim for the opposite arm. Right knee to left arm and left knee to right arm. This one may be a little more awkward or tricky to do, so it may take a bit of practice.

Number 25. Seated Russian Twist (on floor)

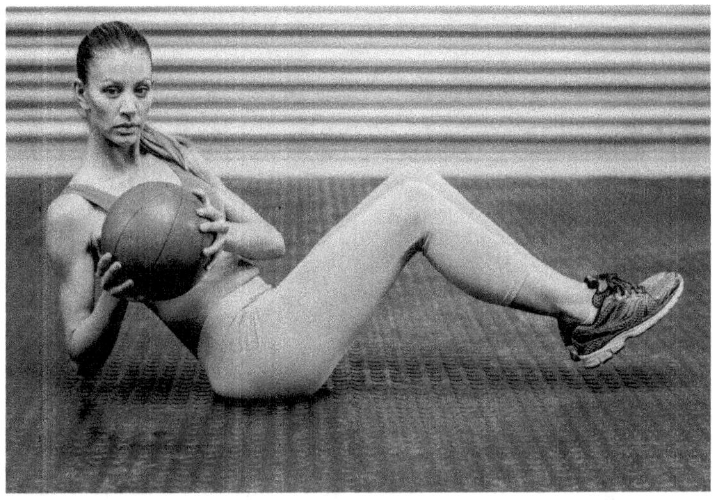

The picture shows a medicine ball being used, but you can do this exercise with or without. It's up to you. If you do not have a strong core to begin with, it would be a good idea to start the Seated Russian Twist without the medicine ball. With your body in somewhat of a V shape and feet off the floor, move your upper body and torso from side to side as if you are going to pick something up on each side of your body.

Number 26. Inner Thigh Leg Lift

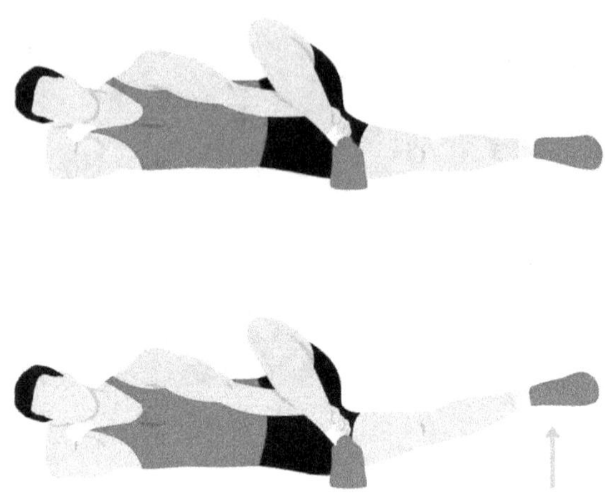

While laying on your side, cross your top leg over your bottom leg and grab your ankle. Move your bottom leg in an upward motion.

Number 27. Pulse Ups

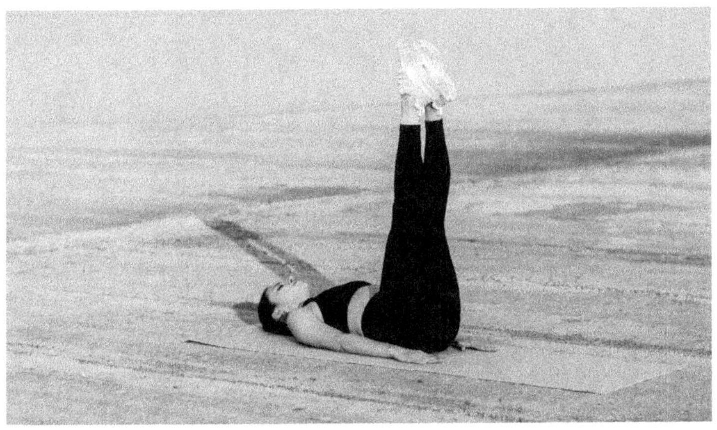

Laying flat on the floor, raise your legs to the ceiling. Lift your butt off the floor and your legs toward the ceiling. You can also place your hands under your butt for a little bit of lift to help things along.

Number 28. Flutter Kicks

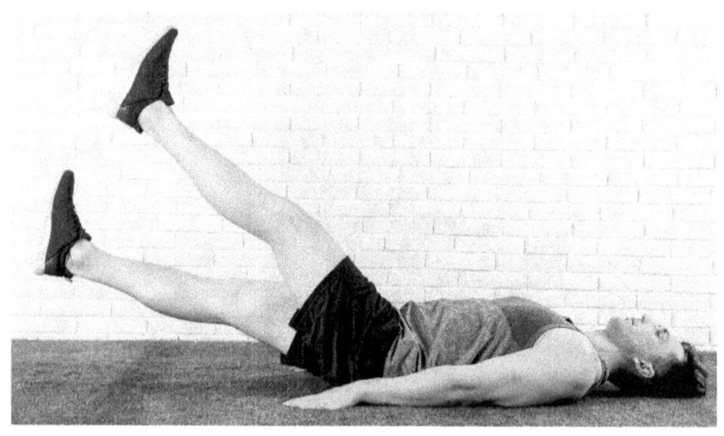

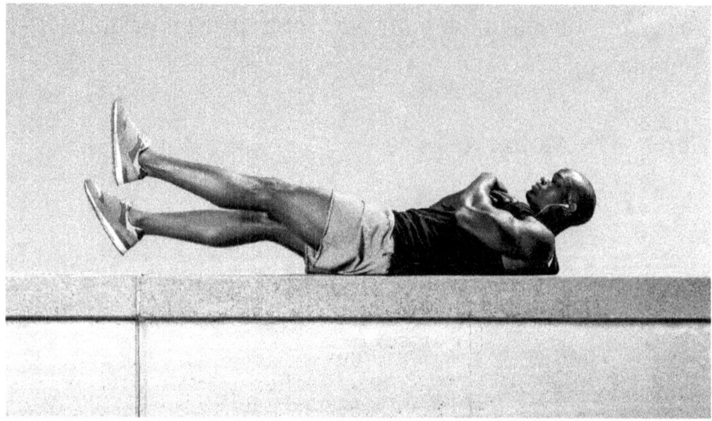

Lay flat on the floor (or retaining wall?) and alternate your legs in an up and down motion. For a variation on this exercise, you can cross your legs back and forth elevating them up and down.

49

Number 29. Windshield Wipers

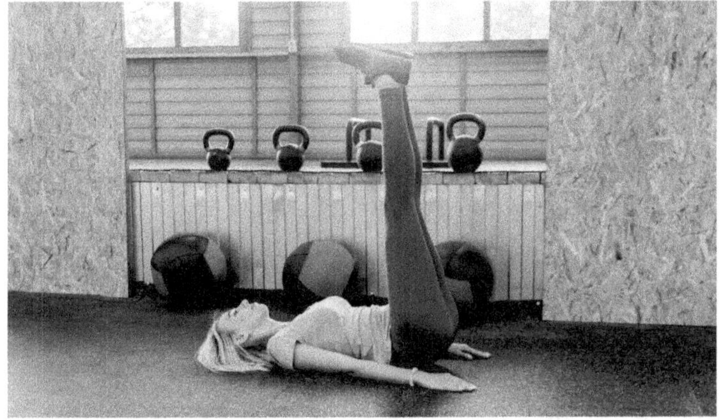

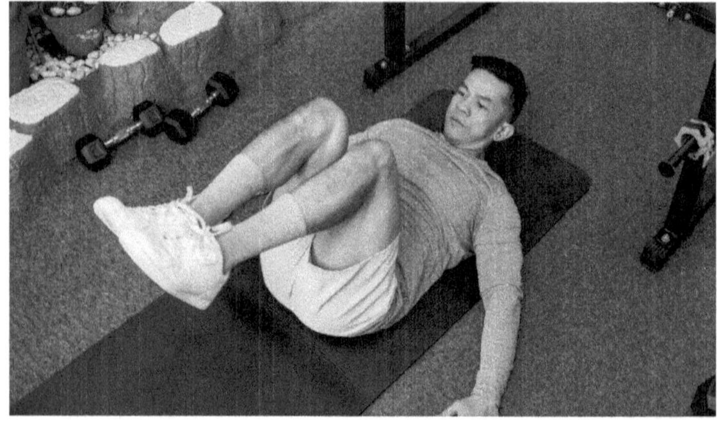

 With your back flat on the floor and your legs raised at either ninety degrees or perpendicular to the floor, move your legs from side to side. This will engage your core. You may need to spread your arms out to afford you some stability while doing this exercise.

Number 30. Modified V Sits

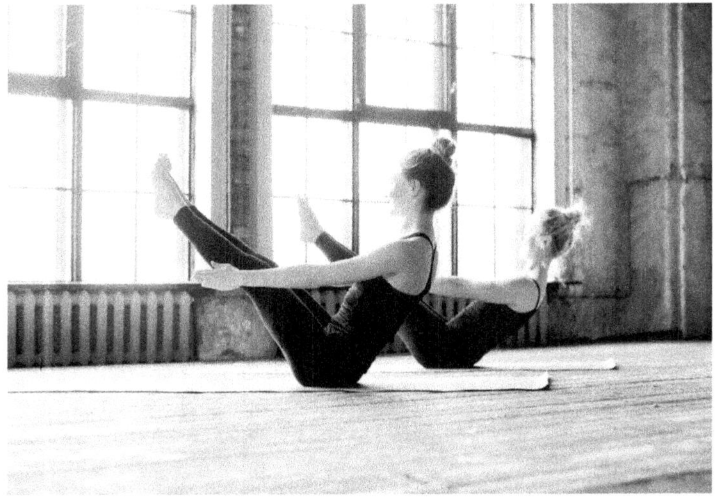

If you are super limber and can sit in this position like the models in the picture, then I applaud you. Most of us will most likely have legs bent if we can balance in this position at all. It certainly takes a bit of practice. As you can see in the picture, the model in the background has a wider position than the model in the foreground. If the wider position is easier for you, it should give you the same results. Hold this position for as long as you can, then relax. Repeat. You can use your hands to stabilize yourself and even "cheat" a bit to help you hold the position. Either way, you will still be engaging your core.

Number 31. Super-man

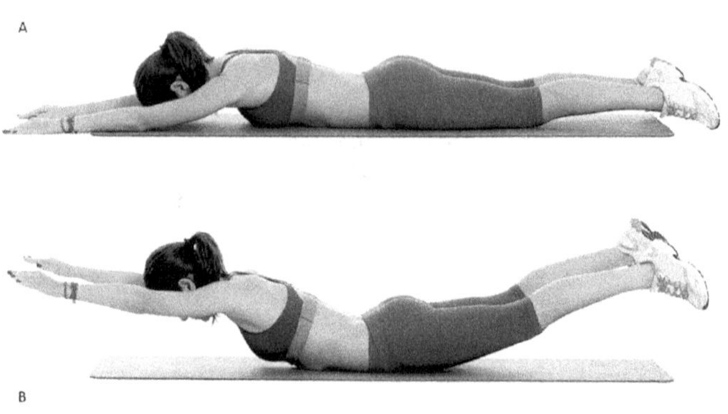

Lay face down on the floor with your arms extended out in front of your head. Raise your arms and legs so your belly and waist are the only parts touching the floor. Hold, then relax. Repeat.

The following exercises employ the use of resistance bands or resistance tube bands/cables with handles. There are pros and cons to each depending on the exercise for which you use them. Resistance tubes or bands can be easily grouped together for increased resistance. There are many different styles and brands out there, so you'll have to do a bit of research to find the ones that will work for you. The resistance tubes with handles offer a bit more flexibility in terms of the exercises you can do with them. It's a great idea to get tubes that come with attachments for use on doors. Just make sure your door is properly closed and strong enough to use in this way if you use these over or under doors.

Number 32. Overhead Press

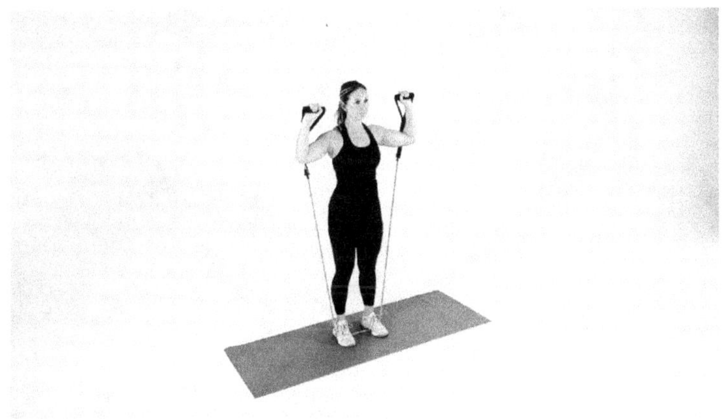

With your resistance tubes with handles attached securely under a door or under your feet, raise the tubes, or bands, to your shoulders. This is your starting point. Begin by pressing the tubes directly above your head and back down. Repeat.

Number 33. Chest Press

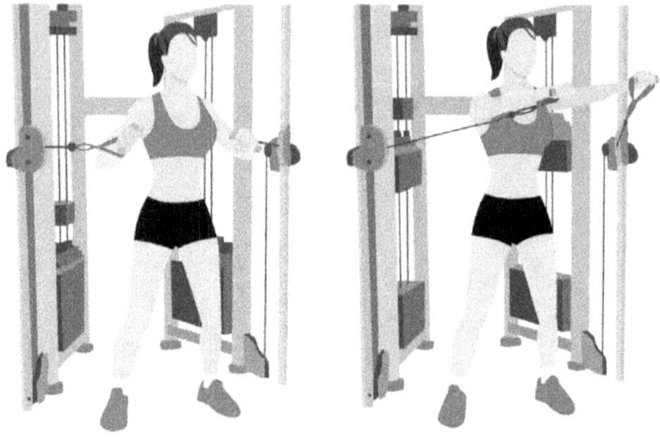

The picture shows a cable machine, but the same principle applies. With your resistance tubes securely attached to the top or bottom of your door, press the tubes outward and away from your chest. Do several reps, then allow yourself to rest a bit, then get more reps in. You can do this Chest Press in a standing position or kneeling position.

Number 34. Standing Tricep Extension

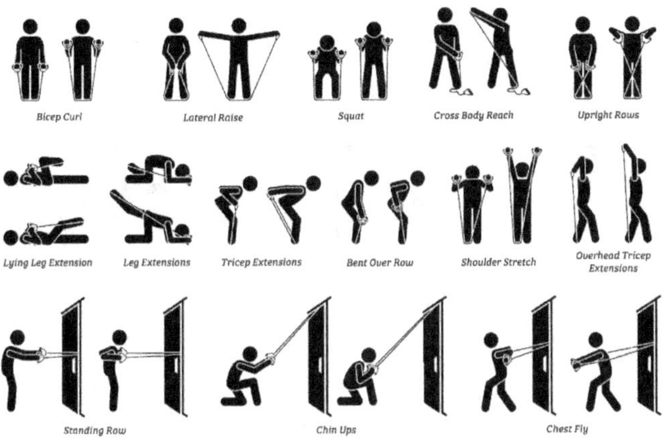

In the picture, locate the "Tricep Extensions" picture. Stand on your bands or tubes. In a sort of skiing position with your knees slightly bent and bending over slightly at the waist, extend your arms behind you and bring back to starting position. Repeat.

Number 35. Bicep Curl

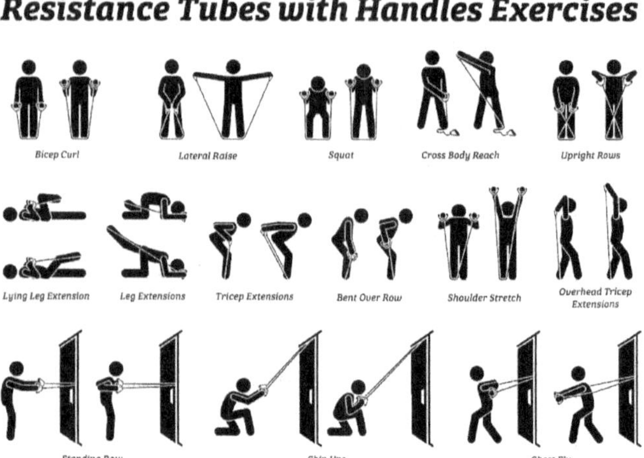

Locate "Bicep Curl" in the picture. While standing on your resistance tubes, bring the tubes to your shoulders and back down. Repeat for several reps.

Number 36. Kneeling Tricep Extension

Resistance Tubes with Handles Exercises

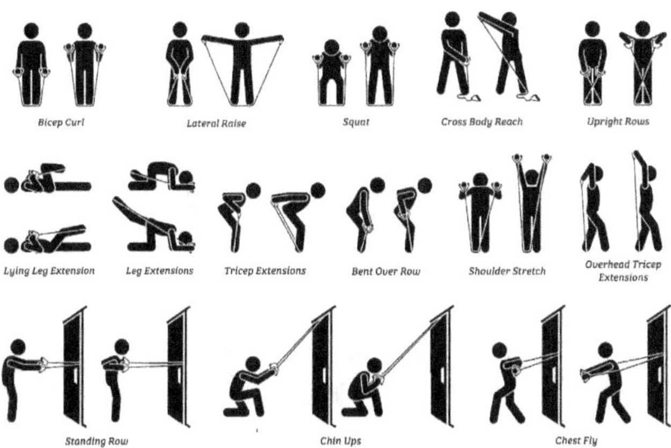

This is similar to the previous "Standing Tricep Extension". But instead of standing, you will be kneeling with the resistance tubes secured underneath the door. While facing the door on your knees, hold the handles down to your side. Move the handles behind your back as far as your arms will allow. Repeat. Please make sure the tubes are tightly secured under your door so they will not slip out from underneath the door and smack you in places you would not prefer. You could seriously injure yourself if the tubes are not secured properly.

Number 37. Standing Overhead Tricep Extension

Resistance Tubes with Handles Exercises

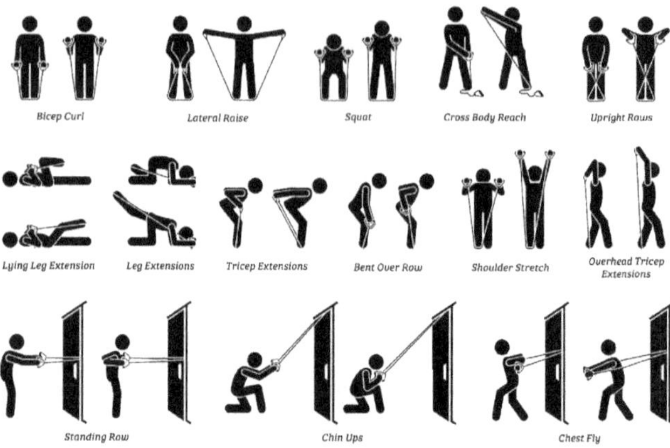

Locate "Overhead Tricep Extensions" in the picture. While standing on your bands or tubes, lift the tubes from behind your head to above your head. Repeat. This will also work if you put the bands under your door. Please note the disclaimer in the previous exercise!

Number 38. Over Door Tricep Pushdown

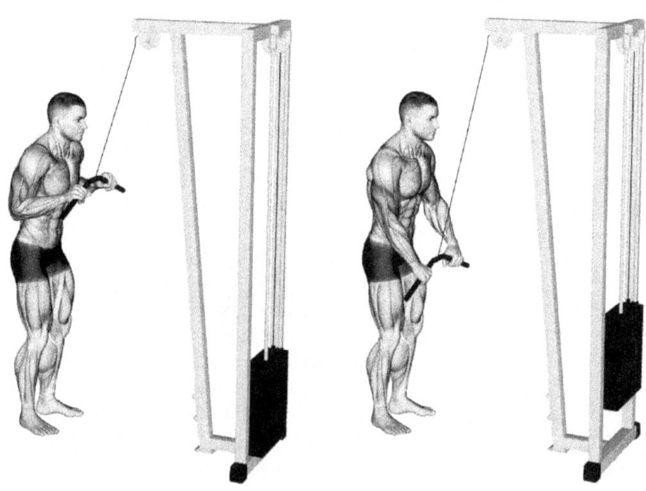

The "model" in the picture is obviously using a cable machine, but the principles of using the resistance bands or tubes still apply. Tightly secure your tube attachment to the top of your door making sure your door is completely closed. You will most likely need to be in a kneeling position to get the best resistance out of the bands. In the kneeling position, the handles will be around chest height. Move them to waist level and back to your sides. Return to the starting position and repeat.

Number 39. Bent Over Row

Resistance Tubes with Handles Exercises

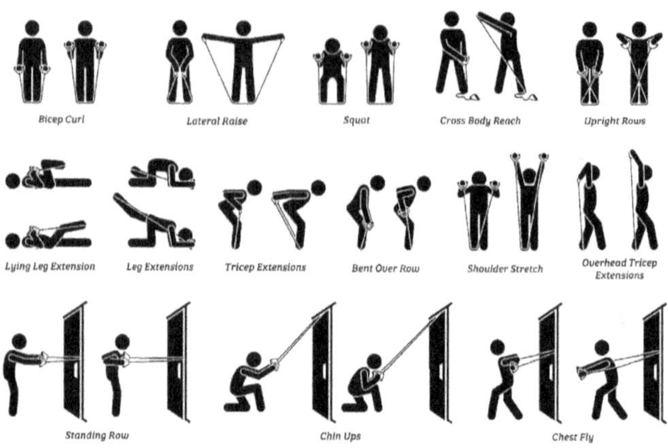

Locate "Bent Over Row" in the picture. Similar to Tricep Extensions, stand on the bands or tubes. With legs slightly bent, pull your handles up your side to where your arms are in a ninety degree position. Return to the starting position and repeat.

Number 40. Feet Wide Apart Squat

Resistance Tubes with Handles Exercises

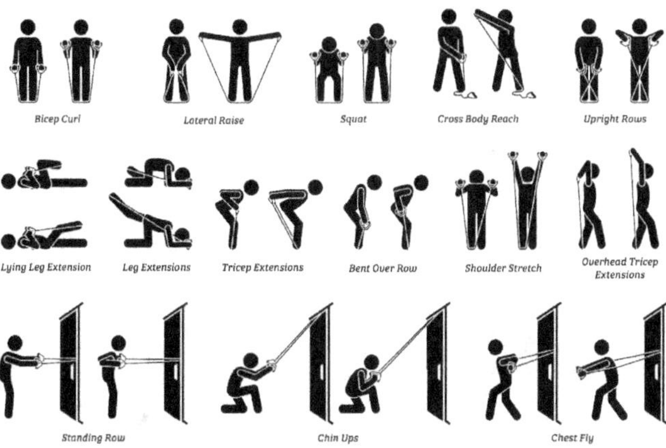

Locate "Squat" in the picture. To obtain the best tension in your bands or tubes, stand with your feet wider than shoulder width apart. Holding your handles or bands with the palms of your hands facing away from you and at shoulder height, perform a squat. Move back to the starting position and begin again.

Number 41. Thruster

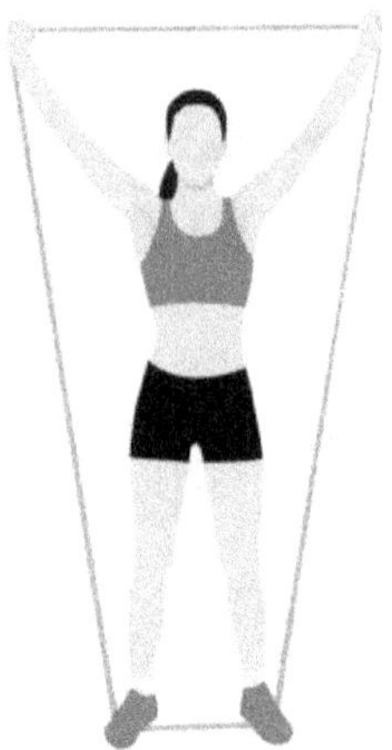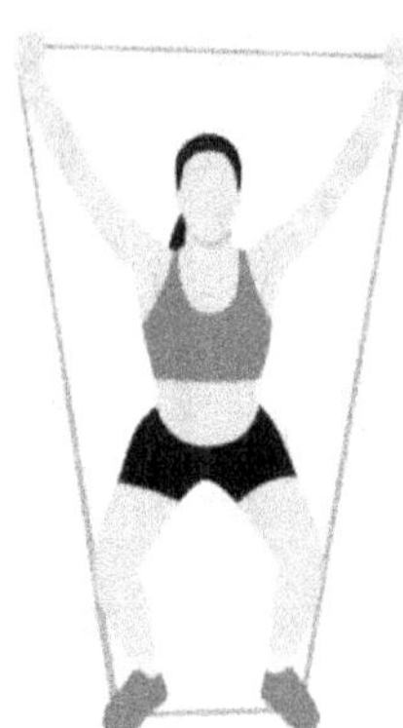

 The Thruster exercise will work your shoulders, arms and legs. Stand on your bands or tubes with feet shoulder width apart and in a squatting position. From the squatting position, stand and raise your bands or tubes over your head with arms extended out and away from your body like in the picture. Move back to the original position and repeat.

Number 42. Lateral Abduction

Resistance Tubes with Handles Exercises

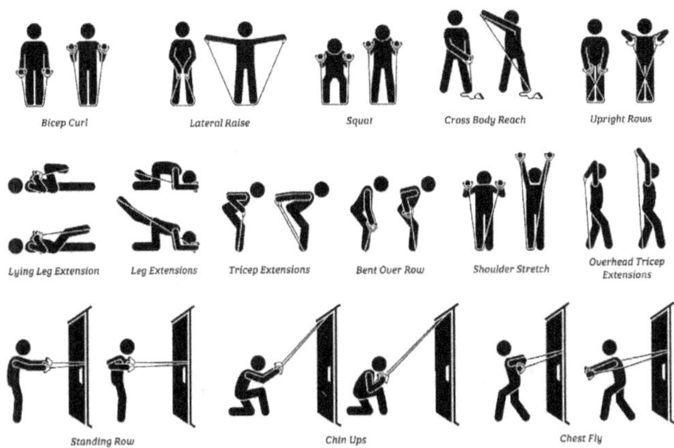

Locate "Lateral Raise" in the picture. While standing on your tubes, raise your arms out to your sides to shoulder height and back down. Repeat. (This is called "abduction" because you are moving your arms away from your body.)

Number 43. Kettlebell Swing

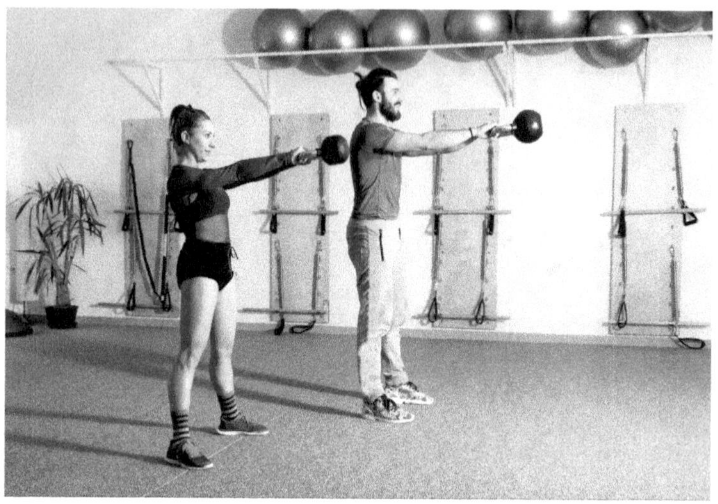

In this exercise, the picture shows kettlebells being used, but you will be using just the resistance bands or tubes. Securely attach the bands or tubes underneath the door. Facing away from the door with the tube between your legs, grab the handle and swing upward. Return to the starting position and repeat.

Number 44. Hip/Leg Abduction

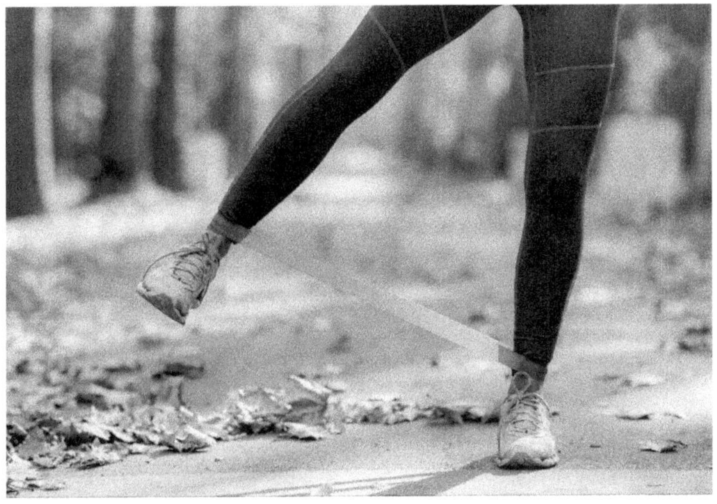

 With your band secured around each foot, or your resistance tubes secured properly underneath your door and to your outside foot, firmly plant your inside foot and move your outside foot away from your inside foot. Bring back to the starting position and repeat.

Number 45. Upright Row

UPRIGHT ROW

WITH RESISTANCE BAND

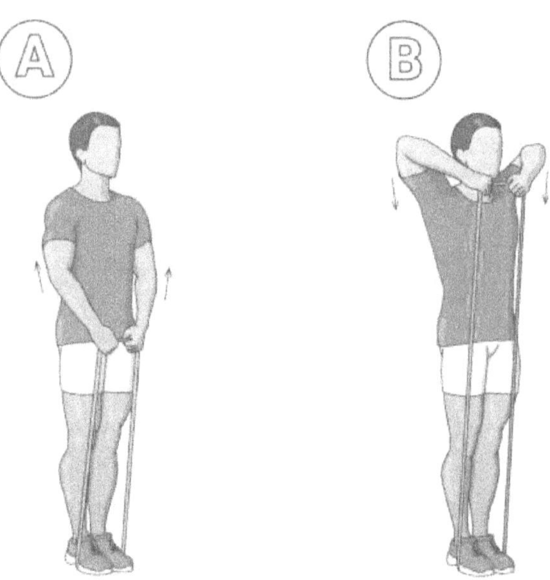

While standing on your resistance bands or tubes, grab the bands or tubes with your palms facing you. Lift up to chin height and back to the starting position and repeat.

Number 46. Face Pull

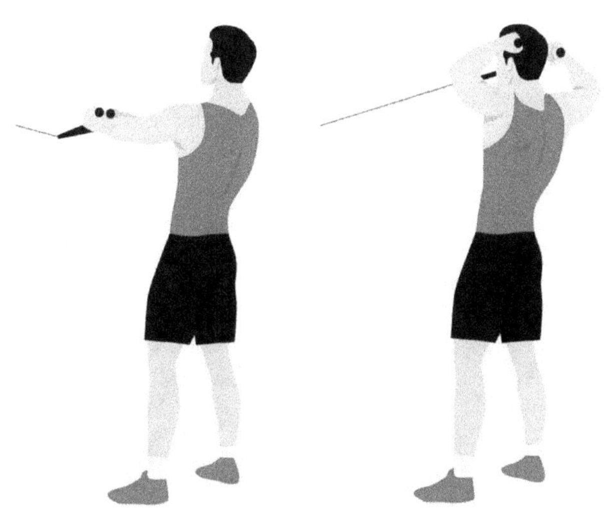

Secure your bands or tubes to the top of your closed door. Facing your door with your arms at shoulder height, pull the band or tubes to your face. Release to the starting position and repeat.

Number 47. Internal Rotation

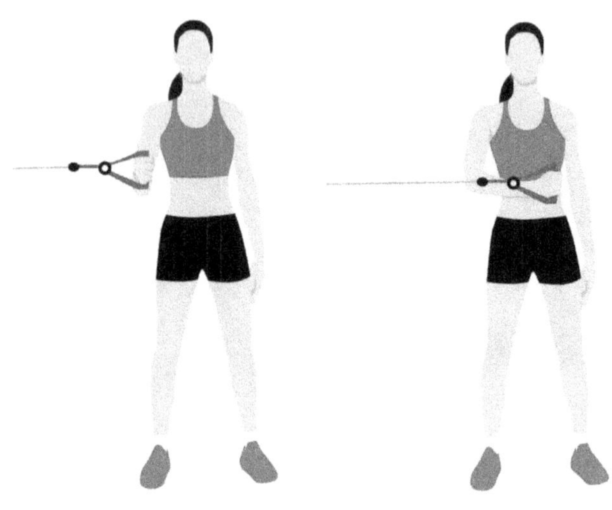

With tubes or bands secured to your door, or whatever fixed, immovable object you have chosen to safely secure your resistance bands, stand with your door to your right or left. With your hand closest to the door, pull the tube across your body. You can keep going and twist your body away from the door and fully extend your arm away from you, or simply return to the starting position and repeat.

Number 48. Vertical Leg Crunch

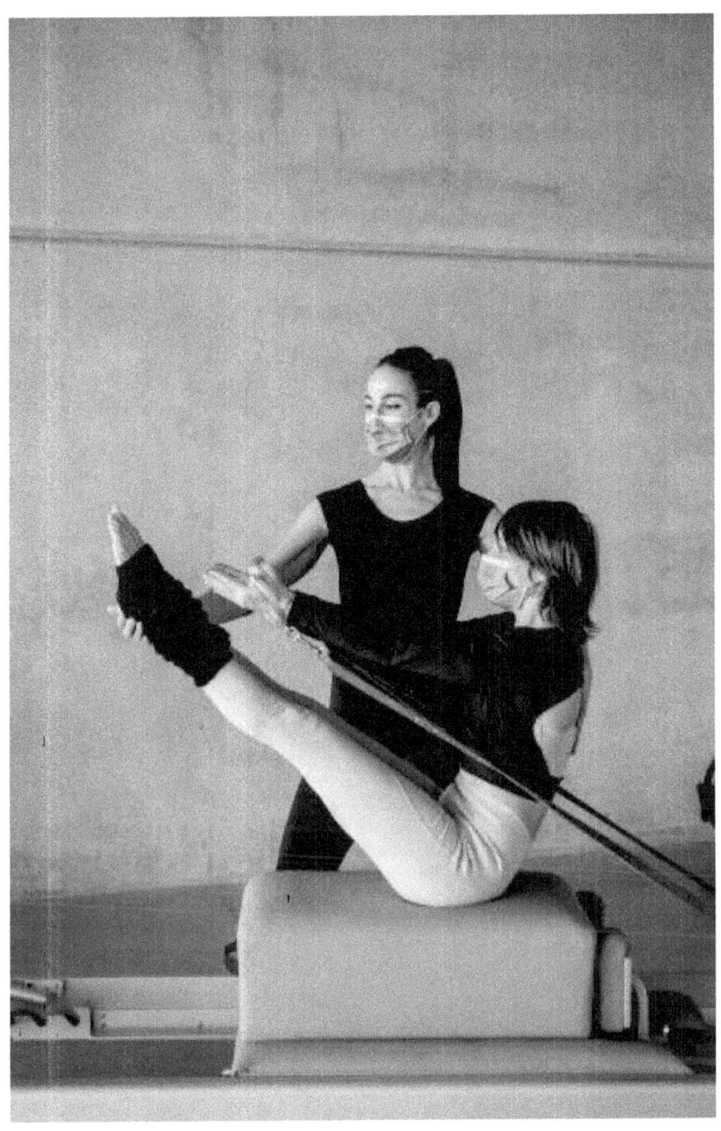

With your resistance tubes secured behind you, lay on the floor or a bench if you have one available. If not, the floor will do just fine. With the bands secured behind you, move to a v sit or crunch position while pulling the bands with you.

Number 49. Kneeling Crunch

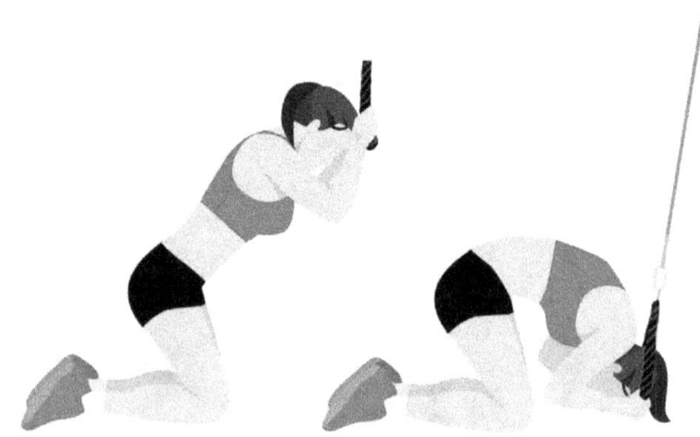

With the resistance tubes secured to the top of your door, in a kneeling position, hold the tubes at forehead level. While holding the tubes in place, move to a face on the floor position. Return to the original position and repeat.

Number 50. Cross Body Reach

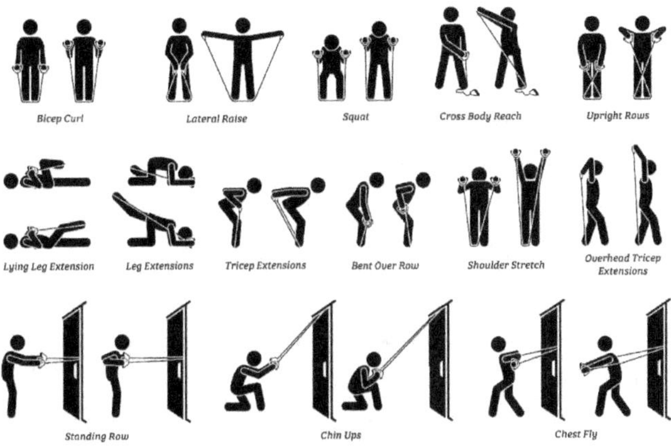

While standing on your resistance tubes or bands with your right foot, use both hands to pull the band from your waist area to above your left shoulder. Return to the original position and repeat. After finishing your reps on that side, move the band to under your left foot. Again, use both hands to pull the band from your waist area to above your right shoulder. Return to the original position and repeat.

Chapter 4

OUTDOOR WORKOUTS

While working out or exercising in the comfort of your own home has its many benefits, spending time outdoors also has a wealth of benefits. There's nothing like fresh air on a nice day. Combine that with walking, running or a good stretch has all the makings of a great day, or a great start to your day. One of my favorite things to do is get up at 5 AM (I know, yuk!) and walk around the track at the park in our neighborhood. It's still completely dark with stars in the sky at 5 AM here. With each trip around the track, which is about a half mile around, I look back to the east and the sky completely changes. I like to see how the sky changes with each trip around the track. If running is your cup of tea, find a safe place to run and have at it. Before running or walking, it's a great idea to get a stretch in. Doing this outside is also a great idea. Taking in the fresh air with a good stretch can really get the oxygen flowing. Muscles feed off oxygen, so get as much fresh air as you can. Whether it's walking, running, biking, swimming, or any other outdoor sport or activity, find time to get outside and enjoy the fresh air.

73

6

Conclusion

I am sure there are a multitude of workouts or exercises not mentioned in this book. Do your research and find the ones that work best for you and your current health and fitness needs. I have listed exercises in this book that have helped me on my journey to lose weight and get stronger. Exercise alone cannot get you to your goal of losing the weight you want to lose. Think of how many years it took you to get you to where you are now. You cannot lose that weight overnight. It will realistically take time. You can make the best, most efficient use of that time by incorporating sensible eating habits into your routine. I am not a nutritionist or a doctor. I also am not a licensed trainer. I only speak from my own experience of achieving my weight loss goals at 51 years old. I wanted to lose my dad-gut and be ripped at 50! I started five months ago and have lost about 30 pounds, so I'm 95 percent to my goal. As far as the ripped part goes, I think I have a two pack. I'll have a six pack before I turn 52 next August. I have not gotten to where I am without sensible, sustainable eating habits centered around portion sizes and eating more foods with low calorie density, as opposed to foods that are high in caloric density. That, along with the exercises in this book, has been the key to my continued success. I am still a work in progress.

I want to thank you for reading Top 50 At Home Workouts! I appreciate your interest in my book and I hope you found valuable information you can use to help you on your road to better health, fitness and well being. I wish you the very best and hope you become your best self. Wow, that sounded cheesy! It's true though, so there ya go.

7

Resources

BOOK COVER

Mayer, S. (2021, December 14). When It Comes To Fitness, Play The Long Game - In Fitness And In Health - Medium. *Medium.* https://medium.com/in-fitness-and-in-health/when-it-comes-to-fitness-play-the-long-game-267d85d55c2d

Wide Hand Push Ups

Durr, D. (2010, April 28). *Big John McHerrman.* Flickr. https://www.flickr.com/photos/dariendurr/4583142780/

Photo #2

Production, S. (2021, July 27). *A couple doing Push-Ups·Free stock photo.* Pexels. https://www.pexels.com/photo/a-couple-doing-push-ups-8933559/

Shoulder With Push Ups

Pixabay. (n.d.). *https://pixabay.com/photos/sport-fitness-e xercise-pilates-1685977/.* Retrieved October 26, 2023, from https://pixabay.com/photos/sport-fitness-exercise-pilates-1685977/

Photo #2

Subiyanto, K. (2020, July 7). *Man in gray tank top doing Push-Ups · Free Stock photo.* Pexels. https://www.pexels.com/photo/man-in-gray-tank-top-doing-push-ups-4720304/

Tricep Push Ups

Lioputra. (2022, July 8). *Woman doing diamond pyramid push ups exercise flat vector. . .* iStock. https://www.istockphoto.com/vector/woman-doing-diamond-pyramid-push-ups-exercise-flat-vector-gm1407479850-458676316?phrase=tricep+push+up&searchscope=image%2Cfilm

Photo #2

Walters, M. (2022, September 22). *This viral TikTok workout is the perfect beginner arm exercise for quick gains.* T3. https://www.t3.com/how-to/viral-tiktok-workout-beginner-arm-exercise

Negative Push Ups

Just use 1st photo from shoulder width push ups -

Pixabay. (n.d.). *https://pixabay.com/photos/sport-fitness-e xercise-pilates-1685977/.* Retrieved October 26, 2023, from https://pixabay.com/photos/sport-fitness-exercise-pilates-1685977/

Ankle Touch Crunches

ARM Systems. (2017, February 6). *Side To Side Ankle Touch*

[Video]. YouTube. https://www.youtube.com/watch?v=yaGb RLJLX5c

Cross Arm Touch Outside Leg Crunches
Porter, A. (2023, July 14). *Add These Four PT-Approved Rotational Exercises To Your Core Workouts.* Coachmaguk. https://www.coachweb.com/exercises/abs-workout/2227/3-step-abs-rotation-exercises

Cross Elbow Crunches
Porter, A. (2023, July 14). *Add These Four PT-Approved Rotational Exercises To Your Core Workouts.* Coachmaguk. https://www.coachweb.com/exercises/abs-workout/2227/3-step-abs-rotation-exercises

Reverse Crunches
McGuire, J., & Hopes, S. (2023, February 16). *How to do a reverse crunch.* Tom's Guide. https://www.tomsguide.com/how-to/how-to-do-a-reverse-crunch

Side Planks
Galic, B. (2023, October 26). *The worst side plank mistakes and how to fix them.* LIVESTRONG.COM. https://www.livestrong.com/article/13727962-side-plank-mistakes/
Photo #2
Nielsen, K. (2020, December 27). *Sportive black woman doing side plank · Free Stock Photo.* Pexels. https://www.pexels.com/photo/sportive-black-woman-doing-side-plank-6303452/

Leg Raise to Reverse Lunge
Dodzy, B. (2020, July 24). *woman in black sports bra and*

black shorts sitting on concrete bench during daytime. Unsplash. https://unsplash.com/photos/woman-in-black-sports-bra-and-black-shorts-sitting-on-concrete-bench-during-daytime-gTTtXwqmKPQ

Photo #2

Fit, C. (2022, August 26). *How to Do High Knees: Benefits, Muscles Worked & Variations.* blog.cult.fit. https://blog.cult.fit/articles/high-knees-exercises-benefits-steps

Wall Sit

Mansuri, M. (2023, August 16). Wall squats can help to lower blood pressure – here's how to perform the exercise at home. *The National.* https://www.thenationalnews.com/lifestyle/wellbeing/2023/08/13/wall-exercises-linked-to-low-blood-pressure-here-are-eight-to-try-at-home/

Squats

Production, M. (2021, May 24). *Photo of a woman in squat position · Free stock photo.* **Pexels.** https://www.pexels.com/photo/photo-of-a-woman-in-squat-position-8032754/

Photo #2

Yodia, R. (2023, August 21). *A man squatting in a park with a ball · Free Stock Photo.* **Pexels.** https://www.pexels.com/photo/a-man-squatting-in-a-park-with-a-ball-18066200/

Plank Leg Lifts

Production, K. (2021, February 3). *Men doing the plank pose one arm leg lift · Free stock photo.* **Pexels.** https://www.pexels.com/photo/men-doing-the-plank-pose-one-arm-leg-lift-6698524/

Photo #2

Shank, M. (2015, December 30). *side plank | RKC School of Strength*. RKC School of Strength. https://rkcblog.dragondoo r.com/tag/side-plank/

Bicycle Crunch

Shvets, A. (2020, October 12). *Ladies doing abs exercise on sports ground · Free Stock Photo*. Pexels. https://www.pexels .com/photo/ladies-doing-abs-exercise-on-sports-ground-5262853/

Photo #2

McGuire, J. (2023c, April 1). I did 100 bicycle crunches a day for a week — here's what happened. *Tom's Guide*. https://ww w.tomsguide.com/news/i-did-100-bicycle-crunches-a-day -for-a-week-heres-what-happened

Reverse Bicycle

Putra, L. (2022c, June 7). *Download Woman doing V sit bicycles exercise. Flat vector illustration isolated on white background for free*. Vecteezy. https://www.vecteezy.com/vector-art/80 56929-woman-doing-v-sit-bicycles-exercise-flat-vector-illustration-isolated-on-white-background

Diver's Push Ups

Group Fitness – Ridge Athletic Clubs. (2023, July 20). Ridge Athletic Clubs. https://ridgeathletic.com/programs/group-fi tness/

Photo #2

Mingorance, J. S., & Sánchez Mingorance, J. (ca. 2023, January). *Woman practicing upward facing dog position at home*. Westend61. https://www.westend61.de/en/imageView/JSMF

02662/woman-practicing-upward-facing-dog-position-at
-home

Burpees

Sudowoodo. (2020, August 2). *Woman doing burpee workout
with pushup, step by step exercise. . .* iStock. https://www.istock
photo.com/vector/woman-burpee-exercise-gm1263390993
-369788837

Mountain Climbers

McGuire, J. (2023b, February 4). I did mountain climbers
every day for a week — here's what happened. *Tom's Guide.*
https://www.tomsguide.com/news/i-did-mountain-climbe
rs-every-day-for-a-week-heres-what-i-learned-about-th
e-ab-exercise

Hip Raise

Production, M. (2021b, July 21). *Woman in Black Top and Pink
Leggings Exercising on the Floor with Fit Ball · Free Stock Photo.*
Pexels. https://www.pexels.com/photo/woman-in-black-to
p-and-pink-leggings-exercising-on-the-floor-with-fit-b
all-8846204/

Single Leg Hip Raise

McGuire, J. (2023b, March 28). I did 50 single-leg glute
bridges for a week — here's the results. *Tom's Guide.* https://w
ww.tomsguide.com/news/i-did-50-single-leg-glute-bridg
es-for-a-week-heres-the-results

Side Plank Leg Lift

https://www.pexels.com/photo/a-woman-doing-a-side-plank-with-one-leg-lifted-4909476/

Photo #2

Shank, M. (2015b, December 30). *side plank | RKC School of Strength*. RKC School of Strength. https://rkcblog.dragondoo r.com/tag/side-plank/

Tricep Dips

Leunen, S. (2020, October 19). *Strong man training in modern gym·Free Stock Photo*. Pexels. https://www.pexels.com/photo/ strong-man-training-in-modern-gym-5496589/

Photo#2

Opolja. (2019, November 4). *Woman exercising working out triceps and biceps doing dips on urban. . . iStock*. https://www.i stockphoto.com/photo/woman-exercising-working-out-tr iceps-and-biceps-doing-dips-gm1184580927-333508168

Tricep Dips Floor

RunMX.com. (2014, January 16). *Fondo de triceps*. Flickr. https://www.flickr.com/photos/runmx/11981572345

Seated Russian Twist

Fit, C. (2022a, July 1). *How to Do Russian Twist for Strong Core: Its Benefits & Variations*. blog.cult.fit. https://blog.cult.fit/a rticles/russian-twists-meaning-how-to-do-correct-form- and-benefits

Inner Thigh Leg Lift

Putra, L. (2022d, December 22). *Download the Man doing Lying Crossover Leg Lift Exercise in 2 steps. Illustration about workout diagram for m. . .. Vecteezy*. https://www.vecteezy.c om/vector-art/16120510-man-doing-lying-crossover-leg-

lift-exercise-in-2-steps-illustration-about-workout-diagr
am-for-muscles-stretch-leg-thing-hip-flat-vector-illustr
ation-isolated-on-white-background

Pulse Ups

Bullmore, H., & Harris-Fry, N. (2023, March 9). *Leg Raises
Are A Great Way To Prevent Lower-Back Pain – Here's How To Do
Them.* Coachmaguk. https://www.coachweb.com/exercises/
abs-workout/172/instant-six-pack-fix-bench-leg-raises

Flutter Kicks

https://www.tomsguide.com/news/i-did-100-butterfly-
kicks-a-day-for-a-week-heres-what-happened

Photo #2

Harris-Fry, N., & Mackenzie, L. (2023, July 21). *How To Do
Flutter Kicks.* Coachmaguk. https://www.coachweb.com/abs-
exercises/8505/flutter-kicks

Windshield Wipers

McGuire, J. (2023c, August 3). *Windshield wipers: How to
do them and the benefits for blasting your core.* Tom's Guide.
https://www.tomsguide.com/how-to/windshield-wipers-h
ow-to-do-them-and-the-benefits-for-blasting-your-core

Photo #2

I did 50 half wipers every day for a week — here's what
happened to my abs. (2023, August 30). *Inkl.* https://www.ink
l.com/news/i-did-50-half-wipers-every-day-for-a-week-
here-s-what-happened-to-my-abs

Modified V-Sit

Howley, E. K., & Bryant, C. X. (2022, June 24). *7 best yoga poses for strength training*. *US News & World Report*. https://health.usnews.com/wellness/fitness/articles/yoga-poses-for-strength-training

Super-man

Exercise like a Superman. (2021, July 27). Good 2 Know El Paso. Retrieved October 29, 2023, from https://good2knowelpaso.org/details/news/exercise-like-a-superman

RESISTANCE BAND EXERCISES

Overhead Press

Band shoulder press. (ca. 2010, January 1). Jefit Workout App. https://www.jefit.com/exercises/445/band-shoulder-press

Chest Press Standing/Kneeling

Putra, L. (2022b, March 12). *Download Woman doing standing cable chest press exercise, Flat vector illustration isolated on white background. Chest workout for free.* Vecteezy. https://www.vecteezy.com/vector-art/6470392-woman-doing-standing-cable-chest-press-exercise-flat-vector-illustration-isolated-on-white-background-chest-workout

Seated Tricep Extension

Resistance tubes band handles exercises stretch workout gym. (2021, March 28). DesignBundles.net. https://designbundles.net/leremy-stick-figures/1284862-resistance-tubes-band-handles-exercises-stretch-wo

Bicep Curl

Resistance tubes band handles exercises stretch workout gym. (2021, March 28). DesignBundles.net. https://designbundles .net/leremy-stick-figures/1284862-resistance-tubes-band- handles-exercises-stretch-wo

Standing Tricep Extension to the Rear

Resistance tubes band handles exercises stretch workout gym. (2021, March 28). DesignBundles.net. https://designbundles .net/leremy-stick-figures/1284862-resistance-tubes-band- handles-exercises-stretch-wo

Standing Overhead Tricep Extension Shoulder and Raise Arms

Resistance tubes band handles exercises stretch workout gym. (2021, March 28). DesignBundles.net. https://designbundles .net/leremy-stick-figures/1284862-resistance-tubes-band- handles-exercises-stretch-wo

Over Door Tricep Push Downs

Ates, D. (2023, August 13). *Strength training exercises — Mr Deniz Ates | Boxing training.* Mr Deniz Ates | Boxing Training. https://www.mrdenizates.com/blog/strength-training-exer cises

Bent Over Row

Resistance tubes band handles exercises stretch workout gym. (2021, March 28). DesignBundles.net. https://designbundles .net/leremy-stick-figures/1284862-resistance-tubes-band- handles-exercises-stretch-wo

Feet Apart Squat

Resistance tubes band handles exercises stretch workout gym. (2021, March 28). DesignBundles.net. https://designbundles .net/leremy-stick-figures/1284862-resistance-tubes-band-handles-exercises-stretch-wo

Thruster

Before you continue. (2022, July 20). Retrieved October 29, 2023, from https://www.google.com/search?q=resistance% 20band%20thruster&tbm=isch&hl=en&tbs=il:ol&sa=X&ved =0CAAQ1vwEahcKEwio95OsjZ2CAxUAAAAAHQAAAAAQAw& biw=1601&bih=894#imgrc=0f0Fvg9RePGi4M

Lateral Abduction

Resistance tubes band handles exercises stretch workout gym. (2021, March 28). DesignBundles.net. https://designbundles .net/leremy-stick-figures/1284862-resistance-tubes-band-handles-exercises-stretch-wo

Kettle Ball Swing

Ayuda, T. (2023, January 29). *What it means if you can't do a kettlebell swing.* LIVESTRONG.COM. https://www.livestrong.c om/article/13776355-cant-do-kettlebell-swing/

Photo #2

Functional training: Just fancy or important? (2022, July 6). Fittr. https://www.fittr.com/article/functional-training-jus t-fancy-or-important-74/

Hip/Leg Abduction

Purdie, J. (2020, March 30). *Resistance band exercises for the inner thigh.* LIVESTRONG.COM. https://www.livestrong.com/article/159448-resistance-band-exercises-for-the-inner-thigh/

Upright Row

Bulgakov, O. (2021, August 28). *Guy Doing Upright Row Home Workout Exercise with Thin Resistance Band. . .* iStock. https://www.istockphoto.com/vector/guy-doing-upright-row-home-workout-exercise-with-thin-resistance-band-or-elastic-gm1336720822-417887647

Face Pull

Putra, L. (2022b, June 27). *Download Man doing cable face pull exercise. Flat vector illustration. Shoulder exercise for free.* Vecteezy. https://www.vecteezy.com/vector-art/8577939-man-doing-cable-face-pull-exercise-flat-vector-illustration-shoulder-exercise

Internal Rotation

Putra, L. (2022b, December 22). *Download the Woman doing External Cable Shoulder Rotation posture for exercise in 2 step. Illustration about. . ..* Vecteezy. https://www.vecteezy.com/vector-art/16138054-woman-doing-external-cable-shoulder-rotation-posture-for-exercise-in-2-step-illustration-about-workout-with-gym-equipment-to-maintain-a-strong-and-stable-shoulder-joint-flat-vector-illustration

Vertical Leg Crunch

Basilico Studio Stock. (2021, April 20). *Woman in protective face mask taking Personal Pilates lesson on a. . .* iStock. https://www.istockphoto.com/photo/young-woman-doing-fitness-pilates-exercise-with-coach-wearing-mask-during-covid-19-gm1306517118-397076532?phrase=vertical+leg+crunches&searchscope=image%2Cfilm

Kneeling Crunch

Putra, L. (2022a, March 9). *Download Woman doing Kneeling cable crunches exercise. Flat vector illustration isolated on white background for free.* Vecteezy. https://www.vecteezy.com/vector-art/6417745-woman-doing-kneeling-cable-crunches-exercise-flat-vector-illustration-isolated-on-white-background

Cross Body Reach

Resistance tubes band handles exercises stretch workout gym. (2021, March 28). DesignBundles.net. https://designbundles.net/leremy-stick-figures/1284862-resistance-tubes-band-handles-exercises-stretch-wo